DOCTORPRENEUR:
Hack Your Growth
With AI And Digital Marketing

**Stop Marketing Struggles, Start Growth
Miracles: Your AI Playbook Awaits**

DR. RISHI V. AACHARYA

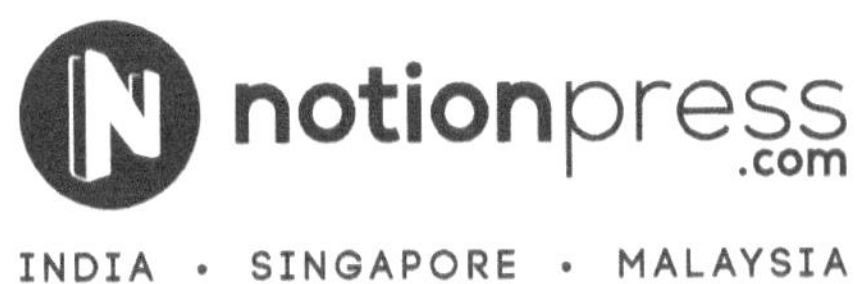

INDIA · SINGAPORE · MALAYSIA

Dedication

To the fallen heroes: the doctors and healthcare workers who selflessly sacrificed their lives during the COVID-19 pandemic, saving countless others.

Your unwavering dedication, courage, and compassion in the face of unimaginable adversity will forever inspire us. This book is dedicated to your memory and the legacy of service you leave behind.

May your sacrifice never be forgotten.

DISCLAIMER

The information contained in this book is for general informational purposes only and should not be construed as the final advice.

While every effort has been made to ensure the accuracy of the information presented, the author and publisher cannot guarantee its completeness or infallibility.

Readers are strongly advised to consult with a qualified digital marketing professional before making any decisions regarding their branding, marketing or advertisement.

The application of any strategies or techniques presented in this book should be tailored to individual circumstances and overseen by a technical and marketing professional.

Neither the author nor the publisher assumes any responsibility or liability for any damages or adverse effects arising from the use of the information contained herein.

Additionally, please note:

- This book is not intended to replace the professional judgment of a digital marketer.

- The information presented may not be applicable to all the healthcare businesses and should be evaluated on a case-by-case basis.

- Digital marketing tools, apps, platforms and methods are constantly evolving, and the information in this book may become outdated over time.

- To maintain the privacy of the clients , I have changed their details such as names, city and practice areas of the doctors in this ebook to give you an example. If it matches anyone, please consider it a pure coincidence.

- While this book includes references to various apps and websites, they are presented for educational purposes only and do not constitute any endorsement. These resources are subject to change by their creators, and readers should use them with caution.

By reading this book, you acknowledge and agree to the above disclaimer

CONTENTS

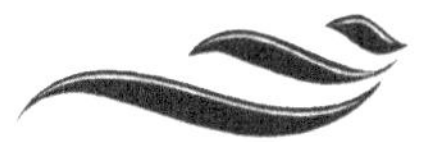

About Me

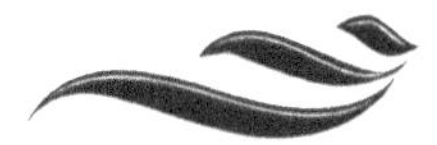

Welcome to the world of **doctorpreneurs**.

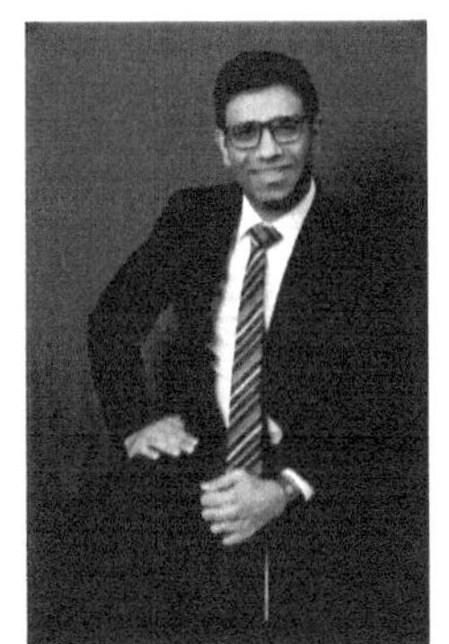

I'm Dr. Rishi Dr. Rishi Aacharya, and I'm here to guide you on your journey to build a thriving healthcare practice, leveraging the power of marketing and technology. With over 13 years of experience in marketing consulting, I've witnessed firsthand the challenges and opportunities faced by healthcare professionals in today's competitive landscape.

My journey began with a deep dive into the world of business at the prestigious Indian Institute of Management Jammu, where I honed my understanding of strategic marketing and growth hacking. Further solidifying my commitment to the field, I became a member of the American Marketing Association, constantly staying updated on the latest trends and best practices. As a growth hacking consultant specializing in the healthcare industry, I've partnered with diverse hospitals and healthcare organizations, helping them unlock their full potential. Through creative and data-driven strategies, I've seen the power of effective marketing in attracting new patients, building loyalty, and ultimately, delivering better healthcare outcomes.

As a growth hacking consultant specializing in the healthcare industry, I've partnered with diverse hospitals and healthcare organizations, helping them unlock their full potential. Through creative and data-driven strategies, I've seen the power of effective marketing in attracting new patients, building loyalty, and ultimately, delivering better healthcare outcomes.

In this book, I share my insights and practical strategies tailored specifically for doctorpreneurs like you. Whether you're starting a new practice or looking to revitalize an existing one, I'm here to guide you through the marketing maze and empower you to achieve your goals.

So, why embark on this journey with me?

- Practical Knowledge: You'll gain actionable strategies and insights drawn from real-world experience, not just theoretical concepts.

- Doctorpreneur Focus: My understanding of the unique challenges and opportunities faced by doctorpreneurs ensures my advice resonates with your specific needs.

- Data-Driven Approach: My strategies are backed by data and proven principles, helping you avoid costly mistakes and make informed decisions.

- Collaborative Spirit: I encourage interaction and questions, fostering a collaborative learning environment where you can tap into my expertise and the collective wisdom of fellow doctorpreneurs.

Ready to unlock the hidden potential of your practice? Dive into this book, embrace the growth mindset, and let's embark on this exciting journey together!

Remember, the success of your practice lies in your hands. Let me be your guide as you navigate the path towards a thriving and fulfilling doctorpreneur journey!

PREFACE

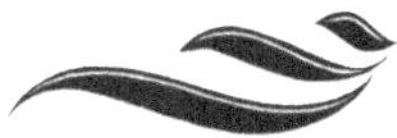

I have known Dr. Rishi Aacharya since a decade now and have actively worked with him on both Strategic and Execution fronts in our flagship SME Training Brand – "Life Champions Ecosystem". During these multiple interactions with him on Online, Offline and Personal levels - I have been in awe of the amazing spectrum of his knowledge - from Spiritual domain on one side, to hardcore Technical domain on the other. He is a Marketing Consultant par excellence, a wonderful Trainer and a valued Mentor to thousands of SME entrepreneurs.

It is very natural that his vast knowledge and experience must come up as a book for the benefit of the world in general and entrepreneurs in particular. In this publication he has focused on Healthcare Professionals/doctors, as this is one busy group where there is maximum dilemma between the business and technical aspects of work. I can vouch that a wide gap has been filled here.

I have observed Dr. Aacharya often stressing heavily on the Mindset of Entrepreneurship which directs 80% of any success, and begins his book from that aspect. As I read the manuscript of this book – I was amazed with the topic layout especially the parts involving the use of AI, social media, advertising and the chapter on embracing the futuristic strategy to stay ahead.

Please use this publication as a reference book. It is not a one-time-read. Neither it is a textbook to be memorized. I will advise you to use it as a reference resource whenever you face business issues or plan on business growth initiatives.

I wish the best for Dr. Rishi Aacharya and for this book to get the deserved attention and success.

Dr Ajay Shesh

P.HD., MBA Marketing, M.Sc. I.T.

Founder – Life Champions Ecosystem & Ajeya Bharat Prakalp

TWO WORDS

WELCOME, DEAR DOCTORPRENEURS!

I recognize the difficulty. Even though you've put your all into growing your medical business, it can be difficult to draw in new clients in the current digital environment. Marketing frequently takes a backseat to scheduling visits, staying current on medical developments, and the never-ending paperwork.

But here's the truth: in today's digital age, a strong online presence is no longer optional, it's essential. Patients search doctors online before making appointments, and if your clinic isn't visible, you're missing out on a vast pool of potential patients.

This is where "Doctorpreneur: Be Your Own Marketing Mastermind with AI" comes into play. Forget outdated marketing tactics and embrace the future with the power of artificial intelligence (AI). This step-by-step guide is your key to unlocking explosive growth for your practice.

But before we dive in, let's talk about your pain points:

- Feeling lost in the marketing jungle? Don't worry, we'll break down complex concepts into actionable steps, tailored specifically for busy doctors like you.

- Drowning in ads and tech jargon? We'll cut through the noise and focus on practical AI tools and resources that are readily available and proven to work for Indian doctors.

- Unsure where to start or how to fit marketing into your already packed schedule? We'll provide a clear roadmap that you can implement at your own pace, even with limited time.

This book is NOT about adding more to your plate. It's about working smarter, not harder. You'll learn how to leverage the power of AI to automate tasks, target the right patients, and skyrocket your online visibility.

Imagine:

- More qualified leads filling your appointment book.

- A thriving online presence that showcases your expertise and builds trust with patients.

- The freedom to focus on what you do best: providing exceptional patient care.

Stop marketing struggles, start growth miracles. Your AI playbook awaits. Let's embark on this journey together and turn you into the Doctorpreneur you were meant to be!

With warm regards,

Dr. Rishi Aacharya

Growth Hacking Consultant For Healthcare Industry

P.S. Don't forget to check out the bonus chapter, checklists, and AI resource recommendations throughout the book. They're your secret weapons for mastering the art of AI-powered marketing!

1

THE DOCTORPRENEUR MINDSET

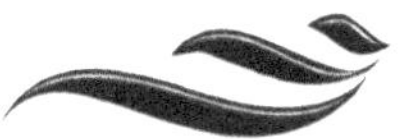

SHIFTING FROM DOCTOR TO DOCTORPRENEUR: EMBRACING THE MARKETING JOURNEY

Congratulations on taking the first step towards becoming a doctorpreneur! Embarking on this path means recognizing that, in today's digital landscape, attracting patients requires a proactive approach. It's about transitioning from a purely clinical mindset to a strategic one, where you don't just see yourself as a healthcare provider, but also as the CEO of your own practice.

However, this shift can be challenging. Let's face it, doctors are wired differently. We're trained to diagnose, treat, and heal, not market ourselves. Yet, here we are, faced with the reality that a robust online presence is no longer optional, it's essential.

But before we dive into the exciting world of AI-powered marketing, let's address the elephant in the room: your limiting beliefs. These are the unconscious thoughts and assumptions that hold you back, often rooted in the following:

1. Fixed Mindset: Believing your abilities and reach are predetermined, leading to statements like "I'm just a doctor, not a salesman." This fixed mindset hinders proactive growth and exploration of new possibilities.

2. Societal Influence: The pervasive idea that doctors should be detached and solely focused on clinical excellence discourages self-promotion and marketing efforts.

3. Common Theories: Misconceptions like "good doctors get patients through word-of-mouth alone" or "marketing is unethical for healthcare

professionals." These outdated notions fail to acknowledge the digital shift in patient behavior.

4. Upbringing and Media: Stereotypes portraying doctors as solely focused on science and devoid of business acumen can solidify limiting beliefs about branching into marketing.

5. Fear of the Unknown: Stepping outside your comfort zone and embracing new tools like AI can raise apprehension about complexity and potential issues.

6. "More Business, More Issues": The misconception that attracting more patients equates to more headaches and administrative burdens, neglecting the potential for better resource allocation and improved efficiency.

These limiting beliefs, while understandable, can act as invisible chains holding you back from reaching your full potential.

The good news? These chains can be broken! Through self-awareness, knowledge, and a willingness to learn, you can shed these limiting beliefs and embrace the doctorpreneur mindset.

Remember, marketing is not about selling yourself; it's about serving your patients better. It's about providing valuable information, building trust, and making yourself accessible to those who need your expertise. It's about taking control of your practice's growth and future.

So, are you ready to embark on this journey? Stay tuned for the next chapter, where we'll delve into the exciting world of AI and how it can empower you to become the doctorpreneur you were meant to be!

TOPIC 2: UNDERSTANDING WHY A STRONG ONLINE PRESENCE MATTERS

As a Doctorpreneur, building a strong online presence is no longer optional – it's essential for your practice's growth and success. But why exactly does it matter so much? Let's explore the key reasons:

1. Online Search by Patients : In today's digital age, over 80% of patients search doctors online before making an appointment. They search for information about your qualifications, experience, expertise, and patient

reviews. If you're not visible online, you're essentially invisible to a vast pool of potential patients.

2. Competition is Increasing: The healthcare landscape is becoming increasingly competitive. More and more doctors are realizing the importance of online marketing, leading to a saturated digital space. Building a strong online presence helps you make a name for yourself in the crowd and attract patients who are actively searching for your services.

3. Build Trust and Credibility: A well-crafted website and engaging social media presence act as digital extensions of your practice. They showcase your expertise, patient testimonials, and valuable information, establishing trust and credibility with potential patients.

4. 24/7 Accessibility: Your online presence never sleeps. It provides patients with convenient access to information about your practice, services, and contact details, even outside of your regular operating hours. This accessibility can be a deciding factor for patients seeking immediate care or information.

5. Improved Communication and Engagement: Online platforms offer valuable tools for patient communication and engagement. You can use email marketing to share educational content, appointment reminders, and special offers. Social media allows for two-way communication, building relationships with patients, and fostering a sense of community.

6. Data-Driven Decisions: Building a strong online presence comes with valuable data and insights. You can track website traffic, analyze patient demographics, and understand what content resonates best. This data helps you make informed decisions about your marketing efforts and optimize your approach for greater impact.

Remember, your online presence is not just a website; it's a dynamic platform that connects you with potential patients, builds trust, and fuels your practice's growth. In the following chapters, we'll explore the practical steps you can take to build a strong online presence, leveraging the power of AI to make the process efficient and effective.

Are you excited to unlock the potential of your online presence? Stay tuned for the next chapter, where we delve into the exciting world of AI and its powerful tools for doctorpreneurs!

TODAY'S PATIENT BEHAVIOR : HOW HE REACHES TO YOU

Gone are the days when a doctor's reputation solely relied on word-of-mouth and proximity. Today's patients are digital-savvy individuals, empowered by information, and actively involved in their healthcare journey. They exhibit the following key behaviors when searching for doctors:

1. Beyond Word-of-Mouth: While recommendations still hold value, patients broaden their search online for diverse perspectives and information beyond their immediate social circle.

2. Proximity : Yes, proximity matters, but online visibility matters More: While location convenience plays a big role, patients are willing to travel further for a doctor with a strong online presence and positive reviews.

3. Reviews and Ratings Rule: Patients scrutinize online reviews and ratings on platforms like Google My Business, Practo, and social media before making an appointment. These reviews act as digital word-of-mouth, shaping their perception of your practice.

4. A doctor's competency is Key: Patients delve deeper into your qualifications, specialization, experience, and past records through your website and online profiles. Highlighting these aspects builds trust and credibility.

5. Personal Testimonials Resonate: Video testimonials and written stories from satisfied patients add a powerful human touch, showcasing your expertise and the positive impact you have on individuals.

6. Infra Photos Create a First Impression: High-quality photos of your clinic's infrastructure, waiting area, and equipment create a positive first impression online. Patients appreciate transparency and a glimpse into the environment they might experience.

7. Warm and Friendly Staff Matters: Positive online mentions of your staff's attentiveness, helpfulness, and overall demeanor foster a welcoming and patient-centric image.

8. Turnaround Time Speaks Volumes: Patients value efficiency and appreciate knowing your average appointment wait time and response time for online inquiries.

9. Follow-up Schedule Shows Care: Demonstrating commitment to post-appointment follow-up through online reminders or patient portals builds trust and ensures continuity of care.

10. Ease of First Interaction is Crucial: Making online appointment booking, virtual consultations, and information acquisition seamless removes friction and improves the patient experience.

Remember, your online presence is a window into your practice. By understanding today's patient behavior and focusing on these key aspects, you can create a positive and informative digital experience that attracts patients, builds trust, and fuels your practice's growth.

Stay tuned for the next chapter, where we explore how AI can empower you to cater to these patient behaviors and optimize your online presence for success!

Overcoming Common Marketing Fears and Excuses: Embracing a Growth Mindset

While understanding the importance of an online presence is crucial, many doctors still harbor fears and anxieties about marketing their practice. Let's address some of the most common ones:

Fear 1: "Marketing feels unethical/inappropriate for doctors."

Remember, ethical marketing focuses on educating patients and providing valuable information, not pushing unnecessary services. You're simply making yourself easily accessible to those who need your expertise.

Fear 2: "I don't have time for marketing; patient care is my priority."

Leveraging AI tools for tasks like content creation, ad management, and social media scheduling can streamline the process, making marketing efficient and time-saving.

Fear 3: "Marketing is too expensive and complicated."

There are plenty of affordable and user-friendly AI tools and resources available specifically for doctors. Starting small and scaling gradually is a viable approach.

Fear 4: "I'm not tech-savvy, and AI sounds intimidating."

Don't worry! This book will guide you through the process step-by-step, breaking down AI concepts into simple, actionable steps. Focus on learning at your own pace.

Fear 5: "What if I make a mistake or say something wrong online?"

Mistakes happen! The key is to be transparent, acknowledge the error, and take steps to rectify it. Building trust and open communication fosters a positive online relationship.

Fear 6: "I'm afraid of negative reviews or online criticism."

Negative reviews, while unpleasant, are sometimes unavoidable. Respond professionally, address the concerns, and use them as an opportunity to improve your practice.

Remember, these fears are often rooted in a fixed mindset. By embracing a growth mindset, you recognize that marketing is a skill to be learned and honed, just like any other medical skill.

Shifting your perspective involves:

- Seeing marketing as an investment in your practice's growth.

- Recognizing the power of AI to simplify and streamline the process.

- Focusing on learning and continuous improvement.

- Developing resilience and accepting that challenges are part of the journey.

By overcoming these fears and adopting a growth mindset, you can unlock the true potential of online marketing and become a Doctorpreneur who thrives in the digital age.

3 Injections of Growth: Learning Attitude, Expert Guidance, and the Experimental Mindset

As you embark on your Doctorpreneur journey, remember: growth doesn't happen in a vacuum. To truly thrive in the digital world, you need three key "injections" into your approach:

1. The Lifelong Learning Attitude:

    The medical field is constantly evolving, and so is the digital landscape. Cultivating a lifelong learning attitude is essential. Embrace new technologies, stay updated on marketing trends, and continuously seek knowledge to refine your digital strategies. Read industry blogs, attend webinars, or enroll in online courses tailored for medical professionals and marketing. Remember, learning is not a sprint; it's a marathon, and every step leads to progress.

2. The Power of Expert Guidance:

While embracing a DIY spirit is commendable, don't hesitate to seek help from experts. Consider collaborating with a digital marketing consultant or agency experienced in the healthcare sector. They can provide valuable insights, create tailored strategies, and guide you through the ever-evolving digital landscape. Remember, you are the expert in your medical field, and external experts can complement your knowledge with specialized marketing expertise.

3. The Experimental Mindset: Embrace "Test & Learn"

The digital world thrives on experimentation and adaptation. Don't be afraid to try new AI tools, explore different marketing channels, and run A/B tests to see what resonates best with your target audience. Track your results, analyze data, and continuously refine your approach based on insights you gain. Remember, every experiment, even if it doesn't yield immediate success, teaches you valuable lessons and fuels future growth.

These three "injections"—(a) a lifelong learning attitude, (b) seeking expert guidance, and (c) embracing the experimental mindset—are your secret weapons for propelling your Doctorpreneur journey. Remember, growth is a continuous process, and by combining your medical expertise with a strategic and open-minded approach, you can build a thriving practice that serves your patients and fuels your passion.

Stay tuned for the next chapter, where we dive into the exciting world of AI and its powerful tools for Doctorpreneurs!

SUMMARY

EMBRACING THE DIGITAL SHIFT:

- Doctors must make the transition from a purely clinical mindset to a strategic Doctorpreneur approach.

- Limiting beliefs like fixed mindsets and societal influences hold doctors back from online marketing.

- A strong online presence is crucial for attracting patients in today's digital landscape.

UNDERSTANDING PATIENT BEHAVIOR:

- Patients search for doctors online before making appointments, looking for qualifications, experience, and reviews.

- Word-of-mouth still matters, but online visibility attracts diverse patients.

- Reviews and ratings significantly impact patient perceptions and decisions.

- Doctor's competency, including qualifications, specialization, and patient experience, is key.

- Personal testimonials and infrared photos create a positive first impression.

- Warm and friendly staff, turnaround time, and follow-up schedules matter to patients.

OVERCOMING MARKETING FEARS:

- Concerns about ethics, time, cost, lack of being tech- savvy, and negative feedback hinder doctor marketing.

- Shifting perspectives and embracing a growth mindset are crucial.

GROWTH MINDSET IN ACTION:

- View marketing as an investment in growth and patient service.

- Embrace lifelong learning and explore AI tools tailored for healthcare marketing.

- Consider seeking guidance from digital marketing experts with healthcare experience.

- Adopt an experimental mindset: try new tools, channels, and A/B Warm and friendly staff, turnaround time, and follow-up schedules matter to patients.

OVERCOMING MARKETING FEARS:

- Concerns about ethics, time, cost, lack of being tech- savvy, and negative

- feedback hinders doctor marketing.

- Shifting perspectives and embracing a growth mindset are crucial.

GROWTH MINDSET IN ACTION:

- View marketing as an investment in growth and patient service.

- Embrace lifelong learning and explore AI tools tailored for healthcare marketing.

- Consider seeking guidance from digital marketing experts with healthcare experience.

- Adopt an experimental mindset: try new tools, channels, and A/B tests for optimal results.

- Track and analyze data to continuously refine your marketing approach.

SELF REFLECTION CHECKLIST

Questions	Yes	No	Notes
Am I ready to Shift from Doctor to Doctorpreneur			
I acknowledge limiting beliefs			
I embrace continuous learning			
I recognize importance of online presence			
I understand Patient Behavior			
I go beyond word-of-mouth referrals			
I consider online reviews and ratings			
I focus on doctor's competency & experience			
I highlight patient testimonials			
I showcase clinic infrastructure photos			
I emphasize warm and friendly staff			
I ensure quick turnaround time			
I offer follow-up schedules			
I simplify the first interaction experience			
I was thinking that marketing is unethical/ inappropriate			
Do I have time for marketing with patient priority?			
Marketing is expensive and complicated			
I am Not tech-savvy and am intimidated by AI			
I have a fear of negative reviews/online criticism			
I view marketing as an investment			
I am open to learning new AI tools and strategies			
I am willing to invest time and resources			

2
THE AI ADVANTAGE: HOW TECHNOLOGY CAN EMPOWER YOU

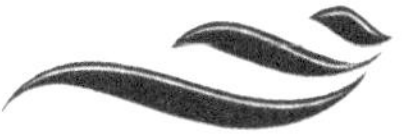

1. DEMYSTIFYING AI: WHAT IT IS AND HOW IT CAN HELP DOCTORS

The world of AI might seem intimidating, but for doctorpreneurs, it holds vast potential to streamline, personalize, and optimize their marketing efforts. Let's break down the complexities and discover how AI can empower you:

WHAT IS AI?

In simpler terms, Artificial Intelligence refers to machines capable of learning and performing tasks typically requiring human intelligence. For doctors, it's not about robots replacing you, but about intelligent tools that augment your capabilities.

HOW CAN AI BENEFIT DOCTORPRENEURS?

While the applications are diverse, here are some key areas where AI can significantly impact your practice:

1. Content Creation: Generate engaging social media posts, blog articles, and email newsletters based on your expertise and patient demographics, saving you valuable time and effort.

2. Personalized Marketing: Analyze patient data and preferences to deliver targeted content and campaigns that resonate with individual needs and interests.

3. Lead Generation and Conversion: Utilize AI-powered chatbots to answer patient inquiries, schedule appointments, and qualify leads, improving engagement and conversion rates.

4. Data-Driven Decision Making: Gain insights from website traffic, social media engagement, and marketing campaigns through AI analytics, helping you optimize your approach for maximum impact.

5. Administrative Efficiency: Utilize AI for tasks like appointment reminders, follow-up emails, and basic administrative duties, freeing up your time for patient care.

Remember, AI is not a replacement for your expertise or human touch. It's a powerful tool that can enhance your existing skills and empower you to serve your patients more effectively in the digital age.

Stay tuned for the next topic, where we delve into specific AI tools and resources tailored for Doctorpreneurs!

2. TOP AI TOOLS AND RESOURCES FOR INDIAN DOCTORS' MARKETING

Navigating the vast world of AI can be overwhelming. Worry not, Doctorpreneurs! Here's a curated selection of top AI tools and resources, specifically tailored for Indian doctors' marketing needs:

CONTENT CREATION:

- Wordtune: Enhance existing content with AI-powered suggestions for grammar, clarity, and tone.

- Pepper Content: Utilize the AI writing assistant to generate blog posts, website copy, and social media content based on your inputs and preferred style.

- Rytr: Generate various content formats like articles, social media captions, and product descriptions tailored to your target audience.

- VidIq: Analyze YouTube video performance and leverage AI insights to optimize titles, descriptions, and thumbnails for greater reach and engagement.

PERSONALIZED MARKETING:

- Pharmeasy Connect: A patient engagement platform utilizing AI to deliver personalized healthcare content and medication reminders.

- Practo Insights: Gain data-driven insights into patient demographics, behavior, and preferences to personalize your marketing campaigns.

- Lybrate Doctor App: Connect with patients, manage appointments, and schedule consultations all within one AI-powered platform.

LEAD GENERATION AND CONVERSION:

- DocSuggest: AI-powered website chatbots answer patient inquiries, qualify leads, and schedule appointments 24/7.

- Zyla Health: Utilize their virtual consultation platform to attract patients, offer online consultations, and collect valuable data.

- ArborVitae Health: Leverage their AI-powered appointment booking system to streamline the process and improve conversion rates.

DATA-DRIVEN DECISION MAKING:

- Google Analytics: Track website traffic, user behavior, and marketing campaign performance with this industry-standard tool.

- Facebook Insights: Analyze social media engagement metrics and gain valuable insights into your audience preferences.

- Practo Reach Insights: Track campaign performance on the Practo platform and tailor your approach for better results.

ADMINISTRATIVE EFFICIENCY:

- DocsApp: Automate appointment reminders, follow-up emails, and patient communication with their AI-powered platform.

- Lybrate Patient App: Streamline appointment scheduling, prescription management, and communication with patients through their app.

- Appointlet: Schedule appointments online effortlessly with AI-powered features and integrations with popular calendars.

Remember, this is just a starting point. Explore these tools, consult with digital marketing experts, and discover innovative solutions that align with your specific practice and needs. As the AI landscape evolves, stay informed and embrace the opportunities it offers to empower your Doctorpreneur journey.

Stay tuned for the next topic, where we delve into crafting a winning website and mastering SEO fundamentals!

3. INTEGRATING AI INTO YOUR EXISTING WORKFLOW: A PRACTICAL GUIDE

Embracing AI isn't about starting from scratch; it's about seamlessly integrating it into your existing workflow to enhance your Doctorpreneur journey. Let's explore practical steps and key considerations:

1. **Identify Repetitive Tasks:**

   Begin by pinpointing repetitive tasks that consume valuable time and effort. These could include:

   - Scheduling appointments: Leverage AI-powered chatbots or appointment booking tools like DocSuggest or Appointlet to automate appointment scheduling and reduce administrative burden.

   - Responding to basic inquiries: Utilize chatbots like Zyla Health or Practo Reach to answer frequently asked questions, provide appointment reminders, and qualify leads, freeing up your time for more complex patient interactions.

   - Generating content drafts: Employ AI writing assistants like Pepper Content or Rytr to create initial drafts for blog posts, social media captions, or email newsletters, allowing you to focus on refining and adding your expertise.

   - Analyzing patient data: Utilize AI-powered tools like Practo Insights or Pharmeasy Connect to gain insights from patient demographics, preferences, and engagement data, helping you personalize your marketing efforts and optimize patient care.

2. **Choose the Right Tools:**

   With numerous AI tools available, prioritize user-friendliness, affordability, and integration with your existing software.

- Consider free trials or demos to ensure the tool fits your needs and workflow before committing.

- Explore tools designed specifically for healthcare professionals, like Lybrate Doctor App or Zyla Health, for seamless integration.

- Look for tools offering API integrations to connect with your existing practice management software or website.

3. **Start Small and Experiment:**

Don't try to integrate everything at once. Choose one or two tasks and experiment with different AI tools to find what works best for you.

- Begin with tasks that have minimal impact on patient care while offering time-saving benefits.

- Track your experience with each tool, noting time saved, efficiency gained, and overall impact on your workflow.

- Don't be afraid to experiment and try different options until you find the perfect fit.

4. **Integrate Gradually:**

Once you've identified impactful tools, gradually integrate them into your workflow.

- Train your staff on using the chosen tools and ensure smooth handovers between AI-powered processes and human interactions.

- Communicate any changes to patients transparently, emphasizing how AI tools enhance their experience and access to care.

- Monitor the impact of AI integration on patient satisfaction and adjust your approach based on feedback.

5. **Prioritize Data Security and Privacy:**

As you navigate the AI landscape, prioritize data security and patient privacy.

- Choose tools with robust security measures and ensure compliance with data privacy regulations like HIPAA.

- Clearly communicate your data usage policies to patients and obtain informed consent before utilizing their information.

- Remain vigilant about data security, and regularly update your AI tools to address potential vulnerabilities.

EXAMPLES OF AI INTEGRATION IN ACTION:

- Dr. Anika, a dermatologist, uses a chatbot to answer basic patient inquiries about appointments, insurance, and clinic hours, freeing up her time for consultations.

- Dr. Rohan, a pediatrician, utilizes an AI content generator to create drafts for his blog posts on child health topics, allowing him to focus on adding his medical expertise and insights.

- Dr. Meera, a psychiatrist, leverages an AI-powered scheduling tool to offer online consultations and manage her appointment calendar efficiently.

Remember, AI is a powerful tool, but it's not a replacement for your expertise or human touch. By integrating AI thoughtfully and strategically into your existing workflow, you can streamline tasks, optimize your practice, and deliver exceptional patient care in the digital age.

Stay tuned for the next topic, where we dive into the exciting world of social media marketing and patient engagement!

SUMMARY

TOPIC 1: DEMYSTIFYING AI:

- AI means machines capable of learning and performing tasks typically requiring human intelligence.

- Benefits for Doctorpreneurs: content creation, personalized marketing, lead generation, data-driven decisions, administrative efficiency.

- Remember: AI augments your skills, not replaces them.

TOPIC 2: TOP AI TOOLS & RESOURCES FOR INDIAN DOCTORS:

- Content Creation: Wordtune, Pepper Content, Rytr, VidIq.

- Personalized Marketing: Pharmeasy Connect, Practo Insights, Lybrate Doctor App.

- Lead Generation & Conversion: DocSuggest, Zyla Health, ArborVitae Health.

- Data-Driven Decision Making: Google Analytics, Facebook Insights, and Practo Reach Insights.

- Administrative Efficiency: DocsApp, Lybrate Patient App, Appointlet.

- Explore, consult experts, and find solutions aligned with your needs.

TOPIC 3: INTEGRATING AI INTO YOUR EXISTING WORKFLOW:

- Identify repetitive tasks: scheduling, inquiries, content drafts, and data analysis.

- Choose the right tools: user-friendly, affordable, and integrated with existing software.

- Start small and experiment: one or two tasks, track experience, and adjust approach.

- Integrate gradually: train staff, communicate changes, and monitor patient satisfaction.

- Prioritize data security and privacy: robust measures, patient consent, and data protection.

SELF ASSESSMENT CHECKLIST

Questions	Yes	No	Notes
I understand the basic principles of Artificial Intelligence (AI) and its potential benefits for my practice.			
I am open to exploring how AI can help me streamline tasks and improve my marketing efforts.			
I am aware of some AI tools and resources specifically designed for healthcare professionals in India.			
I have explored some of these tools and identified a few that might be relevant to my specific needs.			
I am willing to consult with digital marketing experts to learn more about using AI effectively.			
I have identified at least 1-2 repetitive tasks in my workflow that could potentially be automated using AI.			
I am comfortable trying out new AI tools and experimenting with different options.			
I have a plan for gradually integrating AI tools into my existing workflow, considering data security and patient privacy.			
I am prepared to train my staff on using these tools and communicate any changes to patients transparently.			
I am committed to monitoring the impact of AI integration on my practice efficiency and patient satisfaction.			

3

BUILDING YOUR DIGITAL FORTRESS: WEBSITE & SEO BASICS

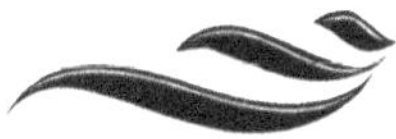

TOPIC 1: CRAFTING A WEBSITE THAT CONVERTS PATIENTS: YOUR ONLINE CLINIC HEADQUARTERS

In the digital age, your website is your online clinic's headquarters. It serves as a crucial platform to showcase your expertise, attract new patients, and build trust with existing ones. This chapter delves into the key elements of crafting a winning website that converts visitors into patients:

FIRST IMPRESSIONS MATTER:

- User-Friendly Design: Ensure your website is easy to navigate with a clear structure, intuitive menus, and search functionality. Patients should find the information they need quickly and effortlessly.

- Mobile-First Optimization: Over 50% of internet searches happen on mobile devices. Make sure your website is responsive and optimized for a seamless mobile experience.

- High-Quality Visuals: Utilize professional photos, videos, and infographics to capture attention, showcase your clinic environment, and build trust.

CONTENT IS KING:

- Publish informative and engaging content like blog posts, patient testimonials, and FAQs to demonstrate your expertise and connect with your audience.

- Tailor your content to your target audience: address their concerns, answer common questions, and highlight your unique selling points.

- Optimize your content for search engines: integrate relevant keywords naturally to improve your website's visibility in search results.

CALLS TO ACTION (CTAS):

- Clearly guide patients towards desired actions: schedule appointments, contact you, or subscribe to your newsletter.

- Place CTAs strategically throughout your website, making them easy to find and visually appealing.

- Track the effectiveness of your CTAs and adjust them as needed based on data insights.

IMPORTANT MENUS AND SUBMENUS FOR A HEALTHCARE WEBSITE:

1. About Us:

   - Importance: Creates trust and familiarity.

   - Key elements:

     - Clinic/Hospital history and mission

     - Team introductions with photos and qualifications

     - Awards and recognitions

     - Virtual tour (this adds a lot of value)

2. Services:

   - Importance: Clearly portrays available services.

   - Key elements:

     - List of services offered with brief descriptions

     - Individual pages for each service with detailed information

     - Fee information (You can give range of your fee)

     - FAQs specific to each service

3. Patients:

   - Importance: Provides crucial information for patients.

   - Key elements:

     - Appointment scheduling options (online, phone, etc.)

     - Insurance information and accepted plans

     - Patient registration instructions

     - Downloadable forms (medical history, etc.)

     - Payment options and billing information

4. Conditions & Treatments:

   - Importance: Educates patients and demonstrates expertise.

   - Key elements:

     - A-Z list of conditions treated

     - Individual pages for each condition, with detailed information

     - Description of treatment options and procedures offered

     - Links to relevant blog posts or articles

5. Resources:

   - Importance: Provides additional value and builds trust.

   - Key elements:

     - Health & wellness articles and blog posts

     - Educational videos and patient testimonials

     - Links to reliable health organizations and resources

     - Treatment Case Studies

     - Downloadable guides

ADDITIONAL IMPORTANT MENUS:

- News & Events: Share clinic news, upcoming events, and community involvement.

- Contact Us: Include all contact information, map, and directions.

- Careers: List open positions and application process.

- Donations: Facilitate donations, if applicable.

Remember:

- User-friendliness: Menus should be clear, concise, and easy to navigate.

- Mobile-optimized: Ensure menus and websites function seamlessly on all devices.

- Search bar: Allow users to easily search for specific information.

- Accessibility: Comply with accessibility guidelines for all users.

- Call to action: Encourage desired actions like appointments or inquiries.

By incorporating these menus and submenus, you can create a user-friendly website that informs, engages, and converts visitors into patients.

BONUS TIPS

CHOOSING A DOMAIN NAME:

- Keep it short, memorable, and easy to spell. Your domain name should be something that people can easily remember and type in their browser.

- Use relevant keywords. This will help people find your website when they are searching for hospitals or clinics in your area.

- Consider using a .com or .org domain extension. These are the most popular and trusted domain extensions for businesses.

- Avoid using hyphens or special characters. These can make your domain name more difficult to remember and type.

- Check for availability. Make sure the domain name you want is not already taken before you register it.

CHOOSING A HOSTING PROVIDER:

- Consider your website's needs. How much traffic do you expect? What features do you need?

- Compare prices and features. There are many different hosting providers out there, so it is important to shop around and find one that meets your needs and budget.

- Read reviews. See what other people have to say about the hosting provider before you sign up.

- Look for a provider with good customer support. You may need help from time to time, so it is important to choose a provider that offers good customer support.

ADDITIONAL TIPS:

- Register your domain name for multiple years. This will help you avoid having to renew it every year and potentially losing it if you forget.

- Use a strong password for your domain name and hosting account.

- Back up your website regularly. This will protect you in case of a data loss.

HERE ARE SOME OF THE POPULAR DOMAIN REGISTRARS AND WEB HOSTING COMPANIES:

- Domain registrars: Google Domains, Namecheap, and GoDaddy

- Web hosting companies: Bluehost, HostGator, and SiteGround

MASTERING THE ART OF SEO: GETTING FOUND BY PATIENTS SEARCHING ONLINE

In today's digital landscape, attracting new patients often hinges on visibility in online searches. Mastering the art of Search Engine Optimization (SEO) empowers you to position your healthcare website at the top of relevant search results, ensuring patients seeking your services easily find you. Here's how to navigate the world of SEO:

Keyword Research: Understanding What Patients Seek

The foundation of SEO lies in identifying keywords and phrases patients use to search for services like yours. Tools like Google Keyword Planner and industry-specific resources can help you uncover relevant keywords with search volume and competition levels. Consider:

- Location-based keywords: Include your city, neighborhood, and nearby landmarks.

- Specific services: Target keywords related to your specialties and procedures offered.

- Patient pain points: Use keywords describing symptoms, conditions, and solutions you provide.

Content Optimization: Providing Value and Relevance

Once you have your keywords, incorporate them naturally into your website content. Remember, valuable and informative content is key to both SEO and patient engagement:

- Create informative blog posts, articles, and FAQs addressing patient concerns and showcasing your expertise.

- Optimize titles, meta descriptions, and headers with relevant keywords but prioritize readability.

- Utilize internal linking to connect related pages within your website, improving user experience and search engine understanding.

- Focus on local SEO: Claim and optimize your Google My Business listing, encourage patient reviews, and cite local directories.

Technical SEO: Building a Strong Foundation

Beyond content, technical aspects play a crucial role in SEO:

- Ensure your website is mobile-friendly: Offer a seamless experience across all devices, as most searches now happen on mobiles.

- Optimize website speed: Fast loading times keep users engaged and improve search ranking.

- Submit your website to search engines: Register with Google Search Console and Bing Webmaster Tools.

- Build backlinks: Earn links from other reputable websites in your field to demonstrate authority and trust.

ANALYTICS AND CONTINUOUS IMPROVEMENT:

SEO is an ongoing process. Utilize tools like Google Analytics to track website traffic, analyze keyword performance, and identify areas for improvement. Adapt your strategy based on data insights and stay updated on evolving search engine algorithms.

REMEMBER:

- SEO is a long-term investment: Results may not be immediate, but consistent effort yields long-term benefits.

- Prioritize patient experience: Don't sacrifice quality content for keyword stuffing.

- Seek professional guidance: Consider consulting with SEO experts for tailored strategies.

By mastering the art of SEO, you can increase your online visibility, attract more patients, and ultimately fulfill your mission of providing exceptional healthcare services.

ADDITIONAL TIPS:

- Leverage social media marketing to further amplify your online presence and engage with potential patients.

- Encourage patient reviews and testimonials on your website and Google My Business listing.

- Run targeted online advertising campaigns to reach specific patient demographics and geographic areas.

I hope this information helps you navigate the world of SEO and position your healthcare practice for success in the digital age!

LOCAL SEO STRATEGIES FOR MAXIMUM VISIBILITY IN YOUR REGION

In today's digital landscape, standing out in your local area is crucial for attracting patients and growing your practice. Local SEO (Search Engine Optimization) specifically targets online searches within your region, ensuring patients actively seeking healthcare services in your vicinity find you easily. Here are some key strategies to boost your local SEO:

CLAIM AND OPTIMIZE YOUR GOOGLE MY BUSINESS LISTING:

- This is your digital storefront, so claim and complete your listing with accurate information like address, contact details, opening hours, and high-quality photos.

- Encourage patient reviews and respond to them promptly, both positive and negative. Positive reviews build trust and improve rankings, while addressing negative ones shows responsiveness and professionalism.

- Utilize the "Services" and "Description" sections to highlight your specialties, procedures offered, and unique selling points.

- Regularly update your listing with events, news, and special offers.

BECOME A LOCAL CITATION HERO:

- List your practice on relevant online directories and websites specific to your region and healthcare field. Popular examples include JustDail, Practo, Lybrate, and local medical association websites.

- Ensure NAP consistency (Name, Address, Phone number) across all listings. Inconsistency confuses search engines and dilutes your local presence.

- Consider paid directory listings for additional visibility in high-traffic directories.

EMBRACE CONTENT MARKETING WITH A LOCAL FOCUS:

- Create blog posts, articles, and guides addressing local concerns and conditions. Target keywords specific to your area and optimize your content for local search.

- Incorporate location-specific elements: mention neighborhoods you serve, local landmarks, and community events you participate in.

- Partner with other local businesses or healthcare providers for guest blogging opportunities. This expands your reach and establishes backlinks to your website.

ENGAGE WITH YOUR COMMUNITY ONLINE:

- Claim profiles on social media platforms popular in your region. Share informative content, respond to comments and messages, and participate in relevant online conversations.

- Consider local online forums and groups related to healthcare or your specific specialties. Share valuable insights and answer questions to build trust and brand awareness.

- Support local events and initiatives, promoting them on your website and social media. This strengthens your community connection and attracts potential patients.

MEASURE AND ADAPT:

- Track your website traffic, analyze local search ranking, and monitor the performance of your local SEO efforts. Tools like Google Analytics and Google Search Console offer valuable insights.

- Adapt your strategy based on data: see what's working well, identify areas for improvement, and adjust your content, keywords, and local outreach accordingly.

Bonus Tip: Encourage patients to leave reviews not just on Google My Business but also on social media platforms and healthcare review websites relevant to their region.

By implementing these local SEO strategies, you can significantly increase your online visibility within your region, attracting more patients seeking healthcare services near them. Remember, consistency, quality content, and active engagement are key to establishing yourself as a trusted healthcare provider in your local community.

GOOGLE MY BUSINESS GUIDELINES FOR CLINICS AND HOSPITALS: PHOTOS, POSTS, REVIEWS, AND LISTING OF SERVICES

Optimizing your Google My Business profile is key for attracting patients online. Here are specific guidelines for each key element:

PHOTOS:

- Number: Use at least 7 photos, showcasing your facility, staff, equipment, and patient experience.

- Quality: Use high-resolution, professional photos that are well-lit and visually appealing.

- Variety: Include photos of the exterior, interior, waiting area, treatment rooms, and relevant equipment.

- Captions: Add captions to each photo, describing what it shows and using relevant keywords.

- Accessibility: Ensure photos are accessible to users with disabilities using alt text descriptions.

POSTS:

- Frequency: Post regularly, ideally 2-3 times per week, to keep patients engaged.

- Content: Share updates, news, events, informative content, special offers, and promotions.

- Visuals: Use high-quality images or videos to grab attention.

- Calls to action: Encourage desired actions like visiting your website, booking appointments, or leaving reviews.

- Scheduling: Schedule posts in advance for consistency.

REVIEWS:

- Importance: Encourage patients to leave reviews, both positive and negative.

- Response: Respond to all reviews promptly and professionally.

- Positive reviews: Express gratitude and show appreciation.

- Negative reviews: Apologize, address concerns, and offer solutions.

- Frequency: Monitor and respond to reviews regularly.

LISTING OF SERVICES:

- Accuracy: Ensure your listed services accurately reflect what you offer.

- Specificity: Use specific names and descriptions for each service.

- Keywords: Include relevant keywords in service descriptions.

- Categories: Choose appropriate categories that match your services.

- Updates: Keep your service list updated as your offerings change.

ADDITIONAL TIPS:

- Follow Google My Business photo and post guidelines.

- Utilize call tracking or UTM parameters to track the effectiveness of your GMB profile.

- Monitor local competitor profiles and see what they are doing well.

- Consider seeking professional help from a healthcare digital marketing agency.

By following these guidelines and staying up-to-date with Google My Business best practices, you can create a strong and engaging profile that attracts new patients and positions your clinic or hospital for success in the digital world.

SUMMARY

- First Impressions Matter: Ensure user-friendly design, mobile-friendliness, and high-quality visuals.

- Content is King: Publish informative and engaging content tailored to your target audience and optimized for search engines.

- Calls to Action (CTAs): Guide patients towards desired actions like appointments, contact, or newsletter subscriptions.

- Important Menus and Submenus: Include sections like About Us, Services, Patients, Conditions & Treatments, Resources, News & Events, Contact Us, Careers, and Donations.

- Bonus Tips: Choose a memorable domain name, use a reputable hosting provider, and register your domain for multiple years.

- Mastering the Art of SEO: Conduct keyword research, optimize content with relevant keywords, focus on technical SEO, and track results for continuous improvement.

- Local SEO Strategies: Claim and optimize your Google My Business listing, become a local citation hero, create local content, engage with your community online, and measure and adapt your strategy.

- Google My Business Guidelines: Use high-quality photos, post regularly, encourage and respond to reviews, and ensure accurate and detailed service listings.

SELF ASSESSMENT CHECKLIST

Questions	Yes	No	Notes
My website has the user-friendly design with clear navigation and search functionality			
My website is mobile-friendly website optimized for seamless experience on all devices			
I have high-quality professional photos showcasing my clinic environment and team			
I have Informative and engaging blog posts, patient testimonials, and FAQs on the website and social media			
My content tailored to my target audience addressing their concerns and highlighting unique selling points			
My content is optimized for search engines with relevant keywords integrated naturally			
I have clear calls to action throughout the website to guide patients towards appointments, contact, or newsletter subscriptions			
I have conducted keyword research to identify relevant patient search terms			
✓ Citations built on relevant online directories and websites in your region			
My Google My Business listing claimed, optimized, and updated regularly with events, news, and special offers			
I have listed on relevant local directories and websites with consistent NAP (Name, Address, Phone number) across all listings			
My website traffic and local search ranking are tracked and analyzed			
My Google My Business profile reviews are being monitored and responded to promptly			

4

CONTENT IS KING: ENGAGING PATIENTS WITH POWERFUL STORIES

In the digital age, understanding the power of content marketing for doctors is crucial for attracting patients, building trust, and establishing yourself as a leading expert in your field. Here's a breakdown of the key benefits:

1. Attract new patients:

    *   Improved Search Engine Ranking (SEO): By regularly creating high-quality, keyword-rich content like blog posts, articles, and FAQs, your website becomes more visible in search engine results, leading potential patients searching for specific conditions or treatments to find you easily.

    *   Build Trust and Authority: Sharing informative and relevant content demonstrates your expertise in your field, building trust with potential patients and positioning you as a reliable source of healthcare information.

    *   Address Patient Concerns: Create content focused on common questions, anxieties, and challenges faced by patients in your specialty. This positions you as someone who understands their needs and provides valuable solutions.

2. Engage Existing Patients:

    *   Stay top-of-mind: Regular content keeps patients informed about your practice, services, and any new developments or treatments

available. This helps maintain engagement and connection even between appointments.

- Promote preventive care: Educate patients about healthy habits and preventive measures related to their conditions, fostering a proactive approach to health management.

- Build a community: Create a platform for interaction and knowledge sharing through comments, forums, or social media groups, fostering a sense of community and support among your patients.

3. Increase Conversions:

- Clear calls to action: Encourage desired actions within your content, such as booking appointments, subscribing to your newsletter, or downloading informative materials.

- Lead generation: Utilize landing pages with targeted content and opt-in forms to capture leads and grow your patient base.

- Patient testimonials: Highlight patient success stories and positive reviews within your content to build trust and encourage others to make appointments.

4. Enhance Reputation and Credibility:

- Establishing Thought Leadership: Share your expertise through blog posts, guest articles, or even online courses, positioning yourself as a thought leader in your field and attracting referrals.

- Positive online presence: Regularly updated, informative content shows patients you're engaged and committed to providing high-quality care, enhancing your online reputation.

- Responding to inquiries and reviews: Proactively addressing patient questions and concerns directly on your content platforms demonstrates transparency and responsiveness, further building trust and credibility.

By understanding the power of content marketing, doctors can leverage its potential to attract new patients, engage existing ones, and create a thriving online presence that supports their practice and ultimately, fosters better patient care.

Remember: Content marketing is a long-term strategy, and consistency is key. Invest in creating high-quality, valuable content that resonates with your target audience, and you'll reap the rewards over time.

CREATING COMPELLING CONTENT THAT EDUCATES AND BUILDS TRUST

In today's digital landscape, patients are increasingly turning to online resources for health information and to choose their healthcare providers. As a doctor, creating compelling content that educates and builds trust is no longer just an option; it's a necessity. Here's your guide to crafting content that resonates with your audience and positions you as a reliable source of information:

UNDERSTAND YOUR AUDIENCE:

- Who are you trying to reach? Analyze your target demographics, their specific needs, and preferred communication channels.

- What are their concerns and questions? Conduct surveys, engage in online forums, and listen to patient feedback to understand their pain points and information gaps.

- What kind of content would be most helpful and engaging for them? Consider video tutorials, infographics, downloadable guides, or interactive quizzes.

FOCUS ON VALUE AND EDUCATION:

- Prioritize accurate, evidence-based information: Cite reputable sources and ensure your content aligns with medical guidelines.

- Address common concerns and misconceptions: Debunk myths and provide clear, understandable explanations of complex topics.

- Offer practical advice and tips: Equip patients with resources to manage their health proactively.

- Share patient success stories: Showcase how you've helped others overcome challenges, building trust and empathy.

CRAFT COMPELLING NARRATIVES:

- Go beyond dry facts and figures: Use storytelling techniques to connect with your audience emotionally.

- Highlight real-life experiences: Feature patient testimonials, case studies, or your own clinical encounters (anonymously).

- Use visuals effectively: Include high-quality images, infographics, and videos to enhance understanding and engagement.

- Maintain a conversational tone: Avoid overly technical language and be approachable and relatable.

OPTIMIZE FOR SEARCH ENGINES:

- Research relevant keywords: Use tools like Google Keyword Planner to identify terms patients are searching for.

- Integrate keywords naturally: Don't stuff your content, but ensure optimal visibility.

- Optimize titles, meta descriptions, and headers: Make them enticing and informative.

- Promote your content strategically: Share it on social media, email newsletters, and relevant online communities.

BUILD TRUST AND TRANSPARENCY:

- Disclose any potential conflicts of interest: Be upfront about sponsorships or affiliations.

- Encourage interaction and ask questions: Respond to comments and messages promptly and professionally.

- Showcase your qualifications and expertise: Link to your professional biography and achievements.

- Highlight patient reviews and testimonials: Let your existing patients do the talking.

REMEMBER:

- Consistency is key: Regularly publish fresh content to maintain audience engagement and improve search ranking.

- Measure and adapt: Track your content performance using analytics and adjust your strategy based on results.

- Seek help if needed: Consider collaborating with healthcare marketing professionals or content creators.

By creating compelling content that educates and builds trust, you can not only attract new patients, but also empower them to make informed decisions about their health. So, put on your writing hat, embrace the power of storytelling, and become a doctorpreneur who guides and empowers your patients through the magic of content!

LEVERAGING AI FOR CONTENT CREATION: STREAMLINE YOUR EFFORTS AS A DOCTORPRENEUR

In today's fast-paced world, doctors often find themselves juggling numerous responsibilities, making content creation for patient education and marketing a daunting task. This is where Artificial Intelligence (AI) emerges as a powerful tool, streamlining your efforts and enabling you to create high-quality content efficiently.

BENEFITS OF AI-POWERED CONTENT CREATION:

- Save valuable time: AI can handle repetitive tasks like keyword research, content formatting, and basic writing, freeing up your time for patient care and other important activities.

- Enhance creativity: AI can suggest new ideas, brainstorm topics, and even generate different writing styles, sparking your creative flow and expanding your content possibilities.

- Personalize content: AI can tailor content to specific patient demographics and needs, making it more relevant and engaging for your target audience.

- Improve accuracy and consistency: AI can ensure factual accuracy and consistency in your content, minimizing the risk of errors and maintaining a professional tone.

- Optimize for search engines: AI can help optimize your content for relevant keywords, improving its visibility in search results and attracting more patients.

EXPLORING AI TOOLS FOR DOCTORS:

- Content generation platforms: Tools like Jasper or Rytr can help you create blog posts, articles, social media captions, and even patient education materials based on your input and desired style.

- Grammar and style checkers: Grammarly and ProWritingAid can help you polish your writing, identify errors, and ensure your content is clear, concise, and professional.

- Keyword research tools: Ahrefs or SEMrush can assist you in identifying relevant keywords and phrases that your target audience is searching for.

- Translation tools: DeepL or Google Translate can help you translate your content into different languages, expanding your reach to a wider audience.

IMPORTANT CONSIDERATIONS:

- AI is a tool, not a replacement: Use it to enhance your content, not create it entirely. Your expertise and personal touch are still crucial for building trust and authenticity.

- Fact-check and edit AI-generated content: While AI is accurate, it's essential to review and ensure the information is factually correct and aligns with your medical expertise.

- Maintain ethical practices: Only use AI tools that adhere to ethical guidelines and avoid generating misleading or harmful content.

- Start small and experiment: Don't overwhelm yourself. Try different AI tools, see what works best for you, and gradually integrate them into your content creation workflow.

Remember: AI is a powerful ally in your Doctorpreneur journey. By using it strategically and responsibly, you can streamline your content creation process, reach a wider audience, and ultimately, empower your patients through valuable and engaging information.

SUMMARY

- Why stories matter: Stories resonate with patients emotionally, build trust, and ultimately drive engagement.

- Types of stories to tell: Share patient success stories, staff profiles, behind-the-scenes glimpses, community involvement, and patient testimonials.

- Crafting compelling stories: Focus on emotions, strong characters, transformation, authenticity, and clear calls to action.

- Platforms for sharing stories: Utilize blog posts, social media, email marketing, website testimonials, and public relations.

- Understanding the power of content marketing: It attracts new patients, engages existing ones, increases conversions, and enhances your reputation.

- Creating compelling content that educates and builds trust: Focus on value, address concerns, use narratives, optimize for search engines, and build trust through transparency.

- Leveraging AI for content creation: AI can save time, enhance creativity, personalize content, improve accuracy, and optimize for search engines.

- Important considerations: Use AI ethically, fact-check content, maintain personal touch, and start small.

Remember: Content marketing is a long-term strategy that requires consistency and a focus on creating high-quality, valuable content that resonates with your target audience. By embracing the power of storytelling and leveraging AI responsibly, you can become a doctorpreneur who empowers patients through the magic of content.

This summary includes the main points from the different sections of Chapter 4 and provides a concise overview of the key takeaways. I hope this is helpful! Let me know if you have any other questions.

SELF ASSESSMENT CHECKLIST

Questions	Yes	No	Notes
I understand the power of storytelling in building trust and engaging patients.			
I am comfortable sharing my own story and the stories of my patients (with their consent).			
I can identify different types of stories relevant to my practice and target audience.			
I regularly create informative and engaging content for my website and social media platforms.			
I focus on addressing patient concerns and providing valuable information in my content.			
I use visuals (images, infographics, videos) effectively to enhance my content.			
I track the performance of my content and make adjustments based on insights.			
I am open to exploring how AI can help me streamline my content creation process.			
I understand the limitations of AI and the importance of maintaining editorial control.			
I am comfortable using AI tools responsibly and ethically.			

5

Social Media Savvy: Engaging with Patients on the Right Platforms

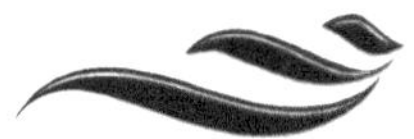

In today's digital age, patients are increasingly turning to social media for healthcare information, seeking connections with providers, and building communities of support. As a doctorpreneur, navigating the diverse landscape of social media platforms can feel overwhelming. But fear not! Chapter 5 equips you with the knowledge and tools to become a "Social Media Savvy" healthcare professional.

This initial topic, "Choosing the Right Social Media Platforms for Your Niche," lays the foundation for your online presence, guiding you towards platforms with the highest potential for reaching the right patients and achieving your unique goals. By understanding your audience, aligning your objectives, and strategically selecting platforms, you can embark on a successful journey of patient engagement and community building through the power of social media. Let's dive in and explore the key steps to choosing the perfect platforms for your niche in healthcare!

Choosing the Right Social Media Platforms for Your Niche

Understanding your audience and presence are crucial steps to selecting the right platform. Here's a guide to navigate the social media landscape:

1. Know Your Audience:

    • Demographics: Age, gender, location, and online habits.

- Needs and concerns: What healthcare questions do they have? What platforms do they frequent?

- Engagement style: Do they prefer short, visual content or in-depth discussions?

2. Define Your Goals:

- Brand awareness: Expand reach and visibility.

- Patient engagement: Build relationships and answer questions.

- Lead generation: Attract new patients to your practice.

- Community building: Create a supportive space for patients.

3. Analyze Available Platforms:

- Facebook: Ideal for general audience engagement, sharing informative content, and running targeted ads.

- Instagram: Highly visual platform, perfect for showcasing your practice through photos and stories.

- Twitter: Real-time news and discussions, suitable for sharing medical updates and engaging in conversations.

- LinkedIn: Professional networking, ideal for connecting with colleagues and showcasing expertise.

- YouTube: Powerful for creating educational videos, patient testimonials, and live Q&A sessions.

- Other niche platforms: Consider physician-specific networks like Doximity or healthcare communities like PatientsLikeMe.

4. Consider Your Resources:

- Time commitment: Each platform requires regular content creation and engagement.

- Team or individual management: Will you handle it yourself or hire a social media manager?

- Paid advertising budget: Consider paid promotions for wider reach and lead generation.

5. Choose Wisely, Start Small, and Experiment:

- Don't be on every platform: Focus on 2-3 where your target audience is most active.

- Start with organic content: Build a foundation before investing in paid advertising.

- Track your results: Analyze engagement metrics and adapt your strategy based on insights.

Bonus Tip: Leverage existing patient feedback and preferences to understand which platforms they favor.

Remember, there's no "one size fits all" answer. By identifying your audience, goals, and resources, you can choose the right social media platforms to connect with patients meaningfully and ultimately achieve your marketing objectives.

CRAFTING ENGAGING SOCIAL MEDIA CONTENT THAT RESONATES

In the previous segment, we explored choosing the right social media platforms for your niche. Now, let's delve into the heart of building a thriving online presence: crafting engaging content that resonates with your target audience. Remember, in the crowded social media landscape, quality and relevance are key to capturing attention and fostering meaningful connections. Here are some essential ingredients for your content recipe:

1. Know Your Audience:

- Go beyond demographics: Understand their online behavior, interests, and pain points related to healthcare.

- Listen actively: Engage in online conversations, respond to comments, and conduct surveys to gather insights.

- Segment your audience: Tailor content to different groups based on their specific needs and preferences.

2. Content Variety is the Spice of Life:

- Mix it up: Utilize diverse formats like images, videos, infographics, blog post snippets, and even live Q&A sessions.

- Educational gems: Share informative content addressing common concerns, debunking myths, and offering practical health tips.

- Patient stories: Showcase success stories, highlight patient journeys, and build trust through real-life experiences (with consent).

- Behind-the-scenes glimpses: Offer a peek into your practice culture, introduce your team, and humanize your brand.

- Humor (used wisely): A touch of humor can be engaging, but ensure it aligns with your professionalism and avoids sensitive topics.

3. Authenticity is the Secret Ingredient:

   - Be yourself and your brand: Let your personality shine through while maintaining professionalism.

   - Transparency is key: Be honest and upfront about your expertise and limitations.

   - Engage in genuine conversations: Respond to comments and messages promptly, fostering a sense of community.

4. Call to Action: The Final Flavor:

   - Clearly state your desired outcome: Encourage website visits, appointment bookings, or content sharing.

   - Make it easy to follow through: Include clear links and instructions.

   - Track and analyze results: Measure engagement and adapt your calls to action based on performance.

5. Consistency is Key to a Winning Recipe:

   - Regularly post content: Develop a content calendar and stick to it.

   - Engage consistently: Respond to comments, participate in discussions, and show your audience you care.

   - Track trends and adapt: Stay updated on platform trends and adjust your content strategy accordingly.

Bonus Tip: Utilize relevant hashtags to increase discoverability and reach a wider audience.

Remember, creating engaging social media content is an ongoing process. Experiment, analyze, and adapt your strategy to keep your audience hooked and ensure your doctorpreneur journey thrives in the social media sphere!

UTILIZING AI TOOLS FOR SOCIAL MEDIA MANAGEMENT AND ANALYTICS

As a busy doctorpreneur juggling multiple responsibilities, managing your social media presence effectively can feel daunting. Fortunately, Artificial Intelligence (AI) emerges as a valuable ally, automating tasks, streamlining workflows, and providing data-driven insights to optimize your social media strategy. Let's explore how you can leverage AI tools to boost your online presence:

1. Content Creation and Scheduling:

   - AI content generators: Tools like Jasper or Rytr can help you create social media captions, post ideas, and even draft informative content based on your chosen topic and style.

   - Image and video creation tools: Platforms like DALL-E 2 or Lumen5 can generate engaging visuals and short videos, saving you time and resources.

   - Social media scheduling tools: Buffer, Hootsuite, and others allow you to plan and schedule your posts across different platforms for consistent presence.

2. Engagement and Community Management:

   - Chatbots: AI-powered chatbots can answer basic questions, address inquiries outside of business hours, and improve overall responsiveness.

   - Sentiment analysis tools: Platforms like Brandwatch or Sprout Social help you understand the sentiment behind audience comments and messages, guiding your communication strategy.

   - Community management tools: Tools like Khoros or Sprinklr help you monitor brand mentions, identify influencers, and manage online conversations effectively.

3. Analytics and Reporting:

    - Social media analytics platforms: Built-in analytics tools or dedicated platforms like Sprout Social provide insights into audience demographics, engagement metrics, and content performance.

    - AI-powered analytics tools: Tools like Socialbakers or Buzzsumo offer deeper insights, identify trends, and predict future performance based on AI analysis.

    - Reporting and optimization: Utilize data insights to understand what's working, identify areas for improvement, and refine your social media strategy.

IMPORTANT CONSIDERATIONS:

- Choose tools that align with your needs and budget: Don't overload yourself with unnecessary features.

- Maintain editorial control: While AI can assist, ensure content aligns with your voice and message.

- Focus on ethical and responsible use: Avoid misleading or harmful content generation.

- Data privacy: Ensure chosen tools comply with data privacy regulations.

Let me remind you here once again that the AI tools are valuable assistants, not replacements. Leverage them to save time, gain insights, and optimize your social media efforts. By combining your professional expertise with the power of AI, you can create a thriving online presence, engage with your audience more meaningfully, and ultimately achieve your Doctorpreneur goals.

SUMMARY

- Choosing the right platforms starts with understanding your audience, niche, and goals.

- Platforms like Facebook, Instagram, Twitter, LinkedIn, and YouTube offer diverse reach and engagement potential.

- Consider resources, team support, and budget for effective social media management.

- Craft engaging content with a mix of formats, valuable information, patient stories, and a touch of personality.

- Be authentic, transparent, and call to action clearly to drive desired outcomes.

- Consistency and adaptation are crucial for long-term success in the social media landscape.

- Utilize AI tools for content creation, scheduling, engagement management, analytics, and reporting.

- Choose AI tools responsibly, maintain editorial control, and prioritize ethical and legal considerations.

SELF ASSESSMENT CHECKLIST

Questions	Yes	No	Notes
I understand my target audience's demographics, needs, and online habits.			
I have clearly defined my social media goals (brand awareness, engagement, lead generation, etc.).			
I have analyzed available platforms like Facebook, Instagram, Twitter, LinkedIn, and YouTube.			
I have considered my time commitment, team resources, and budget for social media management.			
I have chosen 2-3 platforms where my target audience is most active.			
I regularly create diverse content formats like images, videos, infographics, and blog snippets.			
I share informative content addressing common concerns, debunking myths, and offering practical health tips.			
I feature patient success stories and real-life experiences with consent.			
I offer behind-the-scenes glimpses to humanize my brand and team.			
I use humor appropriately while maintaining professionalism.			
I am authentic, transparent, and responsive to comments and messages.			
I include clear calls to action in my content.			
I am open to exploring how AI can help me manage and analyze my social media presence.			
I understand the limitations of AI and the importance of maintaining editorial control.			
I am comfortable using AI tools responsibly and ethically.			
I have evaluated AI tools for content creation, scheduling, engagement management, and analytics.			
I have chosen tools that align with my needs, budget, and data privacy concerns.			

6

PAID ADVERTISING DEMYSTIFIED: REACHING TARGETED PATIENTS ONLINE

Welcome to Chapter 6, where we unlock the secrets of paid advertising for doctorpreneurs! In this first topic, we dive into the two giants of the online advertising world: Google Ads and Facebook Ads. Understanding their capabilities will help you choose the right platform to reach your specific target audience.

1. Google Ads:

- Focus: Reaching people actively searching for healthcare information or specific services.

- Options: Search ads, display ads, video ads, local service ads.

- Strengths:

  - Highly targeted based on keywords and user intent.

  - Reach patients at the crucial moment they're seeking answers.

  - Trackable results and detailed performance insights.

- Weaknesses:

  - Requires ongoing management and optimization for best results.

  - Competitive landscape can lead to higher cost-per-click.

- Best for: Driving website traffic, generating leads, promoting specific services, targeting local patients.

2. Facebook Ads:

- Focus: Reaching a broader audience based on demographics, interests, and online behavior.

- Options: Image ads, video ads, carousel ads, lead generation forms.

- Strengths:

    - Large user base with diverse targeting options.

    - Build brand awareness and engagement beyond active searchers.

    - Cost-effective compared to some Google Ads options.

- Weaknesses:

    - Targeting healthcare services can be restrictive due to regulations.

    - Measuring direct conversions to appointments can be challenging.

- Best for: Building brand awareness, promoting public health initiatives, engaging existing patients, and targeting specific demographics.

CHOOSING THE RIGHT PLATFORM:

- Consider your goals: Are you focused on immediate website traffic or broader brand awareness?

- Know your audience: Where are they most likely to be online? What are their interests?

- Evaluate your budget: How much can you afford to invest in paid advertising?

- Experiment and track results: Test both platforms and analyze data to see what works best.

Remember: Paid advertising is a powerful tool, but it's not a magic bullet. Combine it with organic social media efforts, valuable content creation, and a strong website for a well-rounded online presence that attracts and retains patients.

CRAFTING COMPELLING ADS THAT DRIVE RESULTS

Now that we've explored the different paid advertising options, let's delve into the heart of creating effective ad campaigns that deliver results. Remember, just having an ad doesn't guarantee success. It's about crafting a message that resonates with your target audience and compels them to take action.

1. Define Your Goals and Target Audience:

   - What do you want to achieve? Website visits, appointment bookings, brand awareness, or something else?

   - Who are you trying to reach? Age, location, interests, online behavior, and healthcare needs.

   - Craft a clear buyer persona: Understand their pain points, motivations, and preferred information sources.

2. Craft Compelling Ad Copy:

   - Headline is key: Capture attention with a clear, concise message that speaks to your audience's needs.

   - Benefits over features: Highlight how your service solves their problem, not just what you offer.

   - Urgency and scarcity: Encourage immediate action with limited-time offers or limited spots.

   - Strong call to action: Tell them what you want them to do, clearly and directly.

3. Visual Appeal Matters:

   - High-quality images and videos: Showcase your practice, team, and the value you provide.

   - Relevance to your message: Avoid generic visuals that don't connect with your ad copy.

   - Emotional connection: Use visuals that evoke trust, empathy, and a desire for better health.

4. Landing Page Optimization:

   - Seamless transition: Ensure your landing page aligns with the ad's message and offer.

   - Clear value proposition: Restate the benefits of your service and why they should choose you.

   - Easy conversion path: Make booking appointments, contacting you, or downloading information effortless.

- Mobile-friendly design: A significant portion of users access ads on mobile devices.

5. Targeting and Bidding Strategies:

   - Leverage platform-specific targeting options: Demographics, interests, keywords, behaviors, and more.

   - Start with broad targeting and refine based on performance: Analyze data and adjust your approach.

   - Experiment with different bidding strategies: Cost-per-click, cost-per-acquisition, etc.

   - Track and optimize: Monitor performance metrics and adjust your campaign based on insights.

REMEMBER:

- Compliance is crucial: Adhere to platform regulations and healthcare advertising guidelines.

- Transparency builds trust: Be upfront about your services, pricing, and qualifications.

- A/B testing is your friend: Experiment with different ad variations to see what resonates best.

- Continuous optimization is key. Paid advertising is a dynamic process, so stay adaptable and data-driven.

By following these steps and staying patient, you can create compelling ad campaigns that attract the right patients, drive conversions, and ultimately help your doctorpreneur journey thrive.

AI-POWERED OPTIMIZATION: STREAMLINING YOUR PAID ADVERTISING JOURNEY

In the previous sections, we explored crafting effective ad campaigns and targeting the right audience. Now, it's time to delve into the world of Artificial Intelligence (AI) and how it can further optimize your paid advertising efforts. Imagine having an intelligent assistant constantly analyzing data, suggesting improvements, and making adjustments to ensure you get the most bang for your buck. That's what AI-powered bidding and budget optimization can do for your doctorpreneur journey!

1. Understanding AI in Paid Advertising:

   - AI algorithms analyze vast amounts of data, including user behavior, past campaign performance, and market trends.

   - They predict the likelihood of conversions and automatically adjust bids for each impression in real-time.

   - This allows for highly targeted and efficient spending, maximizing conversions within your budget constraints.

2. Popular AI Bidding Strategies:

   - Target CPA (cost-per-acquisition): Set a desired cost per conversion, and AI optimizes bids to achieve it.

   - Target ROAS (return on ad spend): Define your desired return on investment, and AI optimizes bids for maximum profitability.

   - Maximize conversions: Focus on getting the most conversions possible within your budget.

   - Smart Bidding for Google Search: Google's AI bidding solution, offering various automated strategies.

3. Benefits of AI Optimization:

   - Save time and resources: Let AI handle the heavy lifting of bid adjustments and campaign analysis.

   - Improved campaign performance: AI can achieve better results than manual bidding in most cases.

   - Maximize budget efficiency: Spend your advertising dollars more effectively and reach more qualified patients.

   - Gain valuable insights: AI provides data-driven insights to improve your overall marketing strategy.

4. Important Considerations:

    - Start small and experiment: Don't jump into full AI management immediately. Test it with a portion of your budget.

    - Monitor performance closely: Even with AI, keep an eye on results and adjust strategies as needed.

    - Understand limitations: AI isn't foolproof. Human oversight and strategic guidance are still crucial.

    - Data quality is key: Ensure your targeting and audience data are accurate for optimal AI performance.

5. AI Tools for Budget Optimization:

    - Google Ads Smart Bidding: Built-in AI bidding solution within Google Ads platform.

    - Bing Ads Enhanced CPC: Similar AI bidding option for Bing Ads platform.

    - Third-party tools: Services like Optmyzr or AdEspresso offer advanced AI optimization features.

SUMMARY

KEY TAKEAWAYS:

- Understand platform options: Google Ads & Facebook Ads offer diverse targeting and reach.

- Define goals & target audience: Align campaigns with objectives and ideal patients.

- Craft compelling ad copy: Clear headlines, benefits, strong call to action, emotional appeal.

- Optimize landing pages: Seamless transition, clear benefits, easy conversion path, mobile-friendly.

- Target strategically: Leverage platform options, refine based on performance, experiment with bidding.

- AI for optimization: Automate bidding, maximize budget, gain data-driven insights.

- Start small & monitor: Gradually adopt AI, track results, understand limitations, use high-quality data.

SELF ASSESSMENT CHECKLIST

Questions	Yes	No	Notes
I understand the strengths and weaknesses of Google Ads and Facebook Ads for healthcare marketing.			
I have clearly defined my marketing goals for paid advertising (e.g., website traffic, appointment bookings).			
I have created a detailed buyer persona representing my ideal patient.			
I can write compelling ad copy with clear headlines, benefit-focused messaging, and strong calls to action.			
I use high-quality visuals and videos that are relevant to my ad message and target audience.			
I have optimized my landing pages for seamless user experience, clear value proposition, and easy conversion paths.			
I am comfortable using platform-specific targeting options (demographics, interests, keywords, behaviors).			
I have experimented with different bidding strategies (CPA, ROAS, maximize conversions) based on my goals.			
I regularly monitor and analyze campaign performance metrics (impressions, clicks, conversions, cost).			
I am open to exploring how AI can help me optimize my paid advertising campaigns.			
I understand the limitations of AI and the importance of maintaining control and oversight.			
I am comfortable using high-quality data to ensure optimal AI performance.			

7

Email Marketing Essentials: Nurturing Patient Relationships

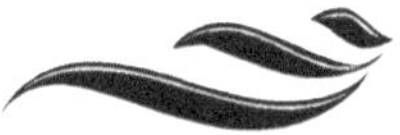

BUILDING AN EMAIL LIST OF ENGAGED PATIENTS

An engaged email list is the lifeblood of successful email marketing for your doctorpreneur journey. It allows you to connect directly with patients, share valuable information, and ultimately, foster stronger relationships that benefit both you and your practice. Let's explore key strategies to build your engaged patient list:

1. Why Build an Email List?

    Before diving in, let's solidify the "why":

    - Direct communication: Bypass social media algorithms and reach patients directly in their inboxes.

    - Targeted messaging: Segment your list for personalized content based on individual needs and interests.

    - Increased engagement: Nurture trust and build long-term relationships with your patients.

    - Promote services and events: Drive website traffic, appointment bookings, and awareness of your offerings.

    - Cost-effective marketing: Reach a large audience for a relatively low investment compared to other channels.

2. Respectful Opt-in Methods:

Building an engaged list starts with gaining consent. Here are some effective methods:

- Website signup forms: Make it easy for patients to subscribe with clear benefits highlighted and GDPR-compliant consent language.

- Patient portal integration: Offer an opt-in checkbox during initial portal registration.

- Business cards and brochures: Encourage signups with QR codes or website URLs prominently displayed.

- In-office signup opportunities: Provide options for patients to join during appointments or check-in processes.

- Social media promotions: Run contests or giveaways, requiring email signups as entry points.

3. Building Trust and Encouraging Signups:

Remember, patients are entrusting you with their inbox. Here's how to build trust and encourage signups:

- Clearly communicate the value proposition: Explain what patients gain by subscribing (e.g., exclusive health tips, appointment reminders, special offers).

- Respect privacy concerns: Emphasize your commitment to data security and adherence to privacy regulations.

- Offer multiple subscription options: Allow patients to choose the content type and frequency they prefer (e.g., monthly newsletters, appointment reminders).

- Use a double opt-in process: Verify email addresses to ensure consent and reduce spam complaints.

- Make it easy to unsubscribe: Include clear unsubscribe links in every email you send.

4. Content is King, Even in Emails:

   Engaged patients stay subscribed to valuable content. Here's how to craft emails that resonate:

   - Informative and valuable content: Share health tips, answer common questions, and promote healthy habits relevant to your practice area.

   - Personalization is key: Use patient names and segment your list for targeted content based on demographics or interests.

   - Maintain a professional and consistent tone: Align with your brand image and ethical guidelines.

   - Clear call to action: Encourage website visits, appointment bookings, or further engagement with each email.

   - Track and analyze results: Monitor open rates, click-through rates, and unsubscribe rates to improve future campaigns.

5. Remember: Building an engaged email list takes time and effort. Be patient, consistent, and provide value to your patients. By following these tips, you can establish a powerful communication channel that nurtures relationships, promotes your practice, and ultimately contributes to your doctorpreneur success.

CRAFTING NURTURING EMAIL SEQUENCES THAT CONVERT: CULTIVATING LONG-TERM PATIENT RELATIONSHIPS

Now that you've built a foundation with an engaged email list, it's time to nurture those relationships and guide patients through their healthcare journey. In this topic, we'll delve into the art of crafting nurturing email sequences that convert—turning subscribers into loyal patients and advocates for your practice.

1. Understanding the Power of Sequences:

   - Beyond single blasts: Sequences deliver a series of connected emails over time, telling a story and fostering deeper engagement.

   - Personalized journeys: Tailor sequences based on patient needs, interests, and actions, offering relevant information and support.

- Nurturing leads to conversions: Guide patients through your funnel, driving website visits, appointment bookings, and ultimately, long-term relationships.

2. Popular Nurturing Sequences for Doctorpreneurs:

- Welcome series: Introduce new subscribers, explain your practice, and offer valuable resources.

- Educational sequences: Address common concerns, provide health tips, and build trust as a knowledge leader.

- Appointment reminder sequences: Reduce no-shows with gentle reminders and helpful information before appointments.

- Post-appointment sequences: Follow up after appointments, gather feedback, and offer ongoing support.

- Seasonal/holiday campaigns: Promote relevant services, educate about seasonal health concerns, and maintain engagement throughout the year.

3. Crafting Compelling Sequence Content:

- Start with clear goals: Define what you want each email in the sequence to achieve (e.g., website traffic, appointment booking).

- Personalize whenever possible: Use names, segments based on demographics or interests, and reference previous patient interactions.

- Offer valuable content: Share informative articles, tips, videos, or case studies relevant to the message and stage of the sequence.

- Include strong calls to action: Clearly tell patients what you want them to do next, whether it's booking an appointment, downloading a resource, or visiting a specific webpage.

- Maintain a consistent brand voice and design: Ensure visual elements and messaging align with your practice's overall branding.

4. Pro Tips for Sequence Optimization:

   - Start simple and experiment: Begin with basic sequences and gradually add complexity based on your comfort level and audience response.

   - Track and analyze results: Monitor open rates, click-through rates, and conversions to see what resonates with your audience and make data-driven improvements.

   - Use automation tools: Leverage email marketing platforms that offer pre-built templates, drag-and-drop sequence builders, and analytics dashboards.

   - Keep it ethical and compliant: Always follow best practices for patient privacy, unsubscribe options, and marketing regulations.

5. Remember: Nurturing email sequences are a powerful tool, but they require consistency and optimization. By understanding your patients, crafting valuable content, and strategically guiding them through their healthcare journey, you can build trust, increase conversions, and establish your practice as a trusted partner in their well-being.

AUTOMATING EMAIL MARKETING WITH AI: SAVE TIME AND MAXIMIZE IMPACT FOR DOCTORPRENEURS

As your doctorpreneur journey takes flight, managing email marketing tasks can become time-consuming, especially when handling a growing list and personalized content. This is where AI (Artificial Intelligence) steps in, offering powerful automation tools to save you time and maximize the impact of your email campaigns. Let's explore how AI can transform your email marketing:

1. Benefits of AI in Doctorpreneur Email Marketing:

   - Personalized content at scale: Leverage AI to dynamically generate personalized subject lines, email greetings, and even content recommendations based on patient data and behavior.

   - Automated segmentation and targeting: AI algorithms can analyze patient demographics, interests, and engagement patterns to automatically segment your list and deliver highly targeted email campaigns.

- Predictive insights and optimization: AI can predict which patients are most likely to engage with specific content or offers, allowing you to tailor your campaigns and maximize conversions.

- Real-time campaign performance analysis: AI continuously monitors and analyzes campaign data, offering real-time insights into open rates, click-through rates, and unsubscribe rates for data-driven optimization.

- Reduced workload and increased efficiency: Automate repetitive tasks like sending reminder emails, scheduling campaigns, and analyzing results, freeing up your time for other crucial aspects of your practice.

2. Popular AI-Powered Email Marketing Tools:

- Klaviyo: Offers AI-powered segmentation, predictive analytics, and personalized content recommendations.

- Mailchimp: Integrates AI for data-driven insights, audience segmentation, and personalized email creation.

- ActiveCampaign: Utilizes AI for smarter segmentation, real-time analytics, and predictive lead scoring.

- HubSpot Marketing Hub: Provides AI-driven email personalization, automated workflows, and predictive lead scoring.

- ManyChat: Leverages AI-powered chatbots for automated patient engagement and personalized email triggers.

3. Getting Started with AI in Email Marketing:

- Identify your goals and challenges: What aspects of your email marketing do you want to automate or improve?

- Choose the right tool based on your needs and budget: Consider features, ease of use, and integration with your existing systems.

- Start small and experiment: Begin with a single AI-powered feature, like personalized subject lines, and gradually expand based on results.

- Focus on data quality and compliance: Ensure your patient data is accurate and adheres to HIPAA regulations for responsible AI use.

- Monitor and analyze results: Track performance metrics and adjust your approach based on data-driven insights.

4. Important Considerations for AI in Healthcare Marketing:

- Transparency and patient trust: Be transparent about using AI and emphasize the benefits it offers patients in terms of personalization and relevance.

- Ethical considerations: Adhere to ethical guidelines for AI use in healthcare and avoid discrimination or bias in your algorithms.

- Human oversight remains crucial: Don't rely solely on AI; maintain human control and judgment in campaign strategy and content creation.

5. Remember: AI is a valuable tool, but it's not a magic solution. Use it strategically, ethically, and in conjunction with your expertise to transform your email marketing, save time, and ultimately, build stronger relationships with your patients.

A COMPREHENSIVE LIST OF TOOLS FOR EFFECTIVE EMAIL WRITING, MARKETING & AUTOMATION WITH TRACKING (WITH LINKS):

Remember: This is not an exhaustive list, and the best tools for you will depend on your specific needs and budget. Consider trying out free trials or exploring platform demos before making a decision.

EMAIL WRITING:

- Grammarly: AI-powered grammar checker and writing assistant (https://www.grammarly.com/)

  - Identifies grammar errors, suggests improvements, and ensures clarity and conciseness.

- Hemingway Editor: Highlights complex sentences, passive voice, and adverbs for better readability (https://hemingwayapp.com/)

- ProWritingAid: Offers advanced grammar checking, style suggestions, plagiarism detection, and a thesaurus for richer vocabulary (https://prowritingaid.com/)

- Mailshake: Provides email templates, personalization features, and A/B testing to optimize engagement (https://mailshake.com/)

- Rytr: AI writing tool generates personalized email copy based on your input, saving time and improving creativity (https://rytr.me/)

EMAIL MARKETING:

- Mailchimp: Is a user-friendly platform for creating campaigns, managing lists, automating workflows, and tracking results (Free plan available) (https://mailchimp.com/)

- ActiveCampaign: Powerful platform with advanced automation, dynamic content, CRM integration, and detailed analytics (https://www.activecampaign.com/)

- Constant Contact: Easy-to-use platform with drag-and-drop builder, segmentation tools, and social media integration (https://www.constantcontact.com/)

- Klaviyo: Ecommerce-focused platform with advanced personalization, predictive analytics, and AI-powered recommendations (https://www.klaviyo.com/)

- HubSpot Marketing Hub: All-in-one platform offering email marketing, landing pages, social media management, and comprehensive analytics (https://www.hubspot.com/pricing/crm)

EMAIL AUTOMATION:

- Zapier: Connects different apps and services, automating tasks like adding subscribers or triggering email sequences (https://zapier.com/apps)

- Pabbly Connect: Streamlines workflows by connecting various apps and services for automated triggers and actions (https://www.pabbly.com/)

- Integromat: Visual automation builder with pre-built workflows for connecting apps and automating marketing tasks (<invalid URL removed>)

- ManyChat: AI-powered chatbot platform that integrates with email marketing for automated patient engagement and personalized triggers (https://manychat.com/)

- Drip: Ecommerce marketing platform with built-in automation for email sequences, abandoned cart emails, and product recommendations (https://www.drip.com/)

TRACKING & ANALYTICS:

- Google Analytics: Tracks website traffic, email campaign performance, and overall marketing effectiveness

- Facebook Insights: Provides detailed analytics for Facebook page performance, campaign reach, and audience engagement

- UTM parameters: Used to track specific sources and campaigns in analytics, understanding where your email traffic originates

- Email marketing platform analytics: Most platforms offer built-in dashboards to track open rates, click-through rates, unsubscribes, and other key metrics.

- Heatmaps and recordings: Visualize user behavior on your emails with heatmaps and recordings to see how your audience interacts

SUMMARY

- Building an Email List of Engaged Patients:

  - Importance: direct communication, targeted messaging, increased engagement, promotion, cost-effective.

  - Opt-in methods: website forms, patient portals, brochures, in-office, social media.

  - Building trust: value proposition, privacy concerns, subscription options, double opt-in, unsubscribe ease.

  - Content is king: informative, personalized, professional, clear call to action, track and analyze.

- Crafting Nurturing Email Sequences that Convert:

  - Power of sequences: personalized journeys, guide through funnel, building trust.

  - Popular sequences: welcome, educational, appointment reminders, post-appointment, seasonal/holiday.

  - Compelling content: clear goals, personalization, valuable content, strong CTAs, consistent branding.

  - Pro tips: start simple, track and analyze, and use automation tools that are ethical and compliant.

- Automating Email Marketing with AI: Save Time and Maximize Impact:

  - Benefits of AI: personalized content, automation, predictive insights, real-time analysis, reduced workload.

  - Popular AI tools: Klaviyo, Mailchimp, ActiveCampaign, HubSpot Marketing Hub, ManyChat.

  - Getting started: identify goals, choose tools, start small, data quality, monitor and analyze.

  - Considerations: transparency, ethical use, human oversight remains crucial.

SELF ASSESSMENT CHECKLIST

Questions	Yes	No	Notes
I have a clear understanding of the benefits of building an email list of engaged patients.			
My website, patient portal, and other materials offer clear and easy opt-in options for email subscriptions.			
I communicate the value proposition of subscribing to my email list and emphasize my commitment to data privacy.			
I offer multiple subscription options to cater to different patient preferences (e.g., frequency, content type).			
I use a double opt-in process to ensure consent and reduce spam complaints.			
I have identified key patient segments and understand their different needs and interests.			
I have developed nurturing email sequences tailored to specific patient segments and goals (e.g., welcome series, appointment reminders).			
My email sequences offer valuable and informative content relevant to each stage of the patient journey.			
My emails include clear calls to action that encourage patients to take the next step (e.g., book an appointment, visit a webpage).			
I track and analyze email performance metrics (open rates, click-through rates, unsubscribe rates) to improve future sequences.			
I am open to exploring the potential of AI to automate and personalize my email marketing efforts.			
I understand the ethical considerations and importance of transparency when using AI in healthcare marketing.			

I have identified specific tasks or aspects of my email marketing that I am considering automating with AI.			
I am aware of and have researched relevant AI-powered email marketing tools that align with my needs and budget.			
I am committed to using AI responsibly and ethically, with human oversight and control over content and messaging.			

8
Measuring Success: Tracking What Matters and Making Adjustments

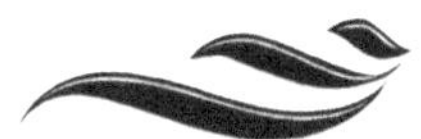

Welcome to Chapter 8, where we delve into the crucial world of Key Performance Indicators (KPIs) for doctor marketing! Tracking the right metrics allows you to understand what's working, identify areas for improvement, and ultimately measure the success of your marketing efforts.

LET'S EXPLORE KEY KPIS SPECIFICALLY RELEVANT TO DOCTOR MARKETING:

1. Website Performance:

    - Website traffic: Number of unique visitors coming to your website, indicating overall reach and patient interest.

    - Page views: Total number of times individual pages are viewed, reflecting content engagement.

    - Bounce rate: Percentage of visitors leaving your website after viewing only one page, indicating potential usability issues.

    - Lead generation: Conversions (e.g., contact form submissions, appointment bookings) generated through your website.

    - Source of traffic: Identify where your website traffic originates (e.g., organic search, social media) to optimize marketing channels.

2. Social Media Engagement:

    - Follower growth: Increase in followers across your social media platforms, reflecting brand awareness and audience interest.

- Reach and impressions: Number of people who see your social media posts, indicating potential impact.

- Engagement metrics: Likes, comments, shares, and clicks on your social media content, showing audience interaction.

- Click-through rate: Percentage of followers who click on links in your social media posts, indicating content effectiveness.

- Sentiment analysis: Gauge the overall sentiment (positive, negative, or neutral) expressed in comments and mentions about your practice.

3. Email Marketing Performance:

   - Open rate: Percentage of recipients who open your email campaigns, indicating initial interest.

   - Click-through rate: Percentage of email recipients who click on links in your emails, showing engagement with specific content.

   - Unsubscribe rate: Percentage of recipients who choose to unsubscribe from your email list, indicating potential issues.

   - Conversion rate: Percentage of email recipients who take a desired action (e.g., book an appointment, download a resource).

   - Email deliverability: Ensure your emails reach recipients' inboxes and avoid spam filters.

4. Patient Acquisition and Retention:

   - Number of new patients: Track new patient acquisition through different marketing channels to identify the most effective ones.

   - Patient acquisition cost: Calculate the cost to acquire each new patient to assess marketing ROI.

   - Patient retention rate: Percentage of existing patients who continue to return to your practice, reflecting patient satisfaction and loyalty.

   - Appointment booking rate: Monitor appointment bookings via different channels to understand patient engagement.

   - Calculate the average revenue a patient brings in over the course of their relationship with your practice.

5. Brand Awareness and Reputation:

- Brand mentions: Track online mentions of your practice name, brand keywords, and doctor names in various channels.

- Sentiment analysis: Analyze the overall sentiment of online mentions to understand public perceptions of your practice.

- Online reviews: Monitor and respond to patient reviews on platforms like Google, Yelp, and Zocdoc, showcasing patient satisfaction.

- Website search ranking: Track your website's ranking for relevant keywords in search engines to gauge organic visibility.

- Media coverage: Track mentions of your practice in local news or relevant publications, boosting brand awareness.

Remember: Choosing the right KPIs depends on your unique marketing goals and patient demographics. Regularly track and analyze your chosen metrics, interpret trends, and make data-driven adjustments to optimize your marketing strategy for ultimate success!

By focusing on relevant KPIs and implementing data-driven decisions, you can gain valuable insights and continuously improve your marketing strategy to attract and retain patients, build a strong brand, and achieve your doctorpreneur goals.

TRACKING YOUR RESULTS WITH GOOGLE ANALYTICS AND OTHER TOOLS

In the previous topic, we explored key performance indicators (KPIs) crucial for measuring your doctor marketing success. Now, let's delve deeper into the tools and platforms that empower you to track these metrics and gain valuable insights:

1. Google Analytics:

- The essential free web analytics tool: Tracks website traffic, user behavior, and campaign performance.

- Monitor key website KPIs: Track page views, bounce rates, source of traffic, and conversions (e.g., appointment bookings).

- Analyze audience demographics and interests: Understand your target audience and tailor your marketing accordingly.

- Set up goals and track conversions: Monitor the effectiveness of specific marketing campaigns in driving desired actions.

- Integrate with other platforms: Connect Google Analytics with your email marketing and social media accounts for unified insights.

2. Social Media Analytics:

- Built-in analytics dashboards: Each social media platform offers native analytics tools to track audience demographics, engagement metrics, and post performance.

- Identify top-performing content: See which posts resonate most with your audience and adjust your social media strategy accordingly.

- Track follower growth and reach: Gauge brand awareness and audience interest over time.

- Measure click-through rates and conversions: Understand how social media contributes to website traffic and other desired actions.

- Analyze sentiment analysis: Gauge public perceptions of your practice through social media mentions.

3. Email Marketing Platform Analytics:

- Dedicated dashboards for email performance: Most email marketing platforms provide detailed analytics on open rates, click-through rates, unsubscribes, and conversions.

- Compare performance across different email campaigns: Identify what resonates best with your audience and optimize your content strategy.

- Segment your email list and track performance by group: Gain insights into specific patient segments and tailor your messaging accordingly.

- Track A/B testing results: Optimize your subject lines, email content, and calls to action based on data-driven insights.

- Monitor deliverability rates: Ensure your emails reach inboxes and avoid spam filters.

4. Patient Relationship Management (PRM) Systems:

- Track patient appointments and interactions: Monitor patient engagement and identify areas for improvement.

- Analyze patient demographics and medical history: Gain insights into your patient base and tailor your marketing accordingly.

- Measure patient satisfaction and feedback: Track patient reviews and feedback to understand their experience and adjust your services.

- Identify marketing leads generated from PRM: Connect marketing efforts with patient acquisition within the system.

- Integrate with other marketing tools: Create a unified view of patient data and marketing performance.

5. Additional Tools for Specific Needs:

- Heatmaps and recordings: Visualize user behavior on your website and emails to understand how patients interact with your content.

- Survey tools: Collect patient feedback and gather valuable insights directly from your audience.

- Online reputation management tools: Track and respond to online reviews across various platforms.

- SEO tools: Monitor your website's search engine ranking for relevant keywords and optimize organic visibility.

- Competitive analysis tools: Benchmark your performance against competitors and identify areas for improvement.

Remember: Choosing the right tools depends on your budget, technical expertise, and specific marketing goals. Start with essential free tools like Google Analytics and social media analytics, and gradually explore paid options as your needs evolve.

By leveraging the power of these tools and tracking the right KPIs, you can gain valuable insights into your marketing effectiveness, identify areas for improvement, and ultimately achieve your doctorpreneur goals of attracting and retaining patients, building a strong brand, and thriving in the digital healthcare landscape.

MAKING DATA-DRIVEN DECISIONS TO OPTIMIZE YOUR DOCTOR MARKETING EFFORTS

So you've collected valuable data through various tools and tracked crucial KPIs. Now, it's time to transform that data into actionable insights that optimize your doctor marketing efforts and drive success. In this topic, we'll explore how to make data-driven decisions and translate insights into effective action:

1. Setting SMART Goals:

    *   Specific: Clearly define your marketing goals, whether it's increasing website traffic, acquiring new patients, or boosting appointment bookings.

    *   Measurable: Ensure your goals are quantifiable so you can track progress and measure success.

    *   Attainable: Set realistic goals that challenge you but are achievable within your resources and timeframe.

    *   Relevant: Align your marketing goals with your overall business objectives and patient acquisition strategy.

    *   Time-bound: Establish a specific timeframe for achieving each goal to maintain focus and drive action.

2. Analyzing and Interpreting Data:

    *   Go beyond raw numbers: Look for trends, patterns, and correlations within your data to uncover deeper insights.

    *   Compare different metrics: Analyze how different marketing channels perform and identify the most effective ones.

    *   Segment your data: Break down your data by patient demographics, interests, or acquisition channels for more specific insights.

    *   Use data visualization tools: Charts, graphs, and heatmaps can help you visualize trends and identify patterns more easily.

    *   Don't ignore negative data: Learn from data that shows what's not working and adjust your strategy accordingly.

3. Taking Action Based on Insights:

- Prioritize areas for improvement: Focus on addressing the biggest opportunities for growth based on your data analysis.

- Develop clear action plans: Define specific steps to implement based on your insights, with responsible timelines and resource allocation.

- A/B tests different approaches: Test variations of your marketing strategies (e.g., ad copy, email subject lines) to see what resonates more with your audience.

- Continuously monitor and adapt: Track the impact of your actions and adjust your approach based on ongoing data and performance trends.

- Communicate results and learnings: Share data-driven insights with your team to encourage a culture of data-driven decision making.

4. Building a Data-Driven Culture:

- Invest in data literacy training: Empower your team to understand and interpret data effectively.

- Encourage data-driven discussions: Foster a culture where data is readily shared, discussed, and used for decision-making.

- Celebrate data-driven successes: Recognize and reward team members who leverage data to achieve positive results.

- Stay informed about industry trends: Keep up-to-date with evolving marketing technologies and data analytics tools.

- Embrace continuous improvement: Continuously learn, adapt, and refine your marketing strategy based on data-driven insights.

Remember: Implementing a data-driven approach is an ongoing process, not a one-time effort. By setting SMART goals, analyzing data effectively, taking action based on insights, and building a data-driven culture, you can unlock the true potential of your doctor marketing efforts and achieve sustainable success in the digital healthcare landscape.

By embracing data as a powerful partner, you can navigate the evolving healthcare landscape with confidence and make informed decisions that attract and retain patients, build trust, and achieve your doctorpreneur goals.

SUMMARY

- Website performance: traffic, page views, bounce rate, lead generation, source of traffic.

- Social media engagement: follower growth, reach, impressions, clicks, sentiment analysis.

- Email marketing performance: open rate, click-through rate, unsubscribe rate, conversion rate, deliverability.

- Patient acquisition and retention: new patients, acquisition cost, retention rate, appointment booking rate, lifetime value.

- Brand awareness and reputation: mentions, sentiment analysis, online reviews, website search ranking, media coverage.

- Google Analytics: free tool for website traffic, user behavior, and campaign performance.

- Social media analytics: track audience demographics, engagement, and post performance.

- Email marketing platform analytics: monitor open rates, clicks, unsubscribes, and conversions.

- Patient Relationship Management (PRM) systems: track appointments, patient data, feedback, and marketing leads.

- Additional tools: heatmaps, surveys, reputation management, SEO tools, competitive analysis.

- Set SMART goals: specific, measurable, attainable, relevant, and time-bound.

- Analyze and interpret data: find trends, patterns, segment data, use visualization tools.

- Take action based on insights: prioritize improvements, develop action plans, A/B test, monitor, and adapt.

- Build a data-driven culture: invest in training, encourage discussions, celebrate successes, stay informed, and embrace continuous improvement.

SELF ASSESSMENT CHECKLIST

Questions	Yes	No	Notes
I have clearly defined SMART goals for my doctor marketing efforts.			
My goals are aligned with my overall business objectives and patient acquisition strategy.			
I have established specific timeframes for achieving each of my goals.			
Tracking Key Performance Indicators (KPIs)			
I am tracking relevant KPIs that align with my marketing goals (e.g., website traffic, patient acquisition, brand awareness).			
I am using appropriate tools and platforms to track my chosen KPIs (e.g., Google Analytics, social media analytics, email marketing platform analytics).			
I am regularly monitoring and analyzing my KPI data to identify trends and patterns.			
I am actively using data insights to inform my marketing decisions and strategy adjustments.			
I am able to identify areas for improvement based on my data analysis.			
I am developing and implementing clear action plans based on my data-driven insights.			
I am regularly testing different approaches and measuring their effectiveness using A/B testing or similar methods.			

I am encouraging my team to be more data-literate and understand the importance of data analysis.			
We regularly discuss and share data insights within the team to inform decision-making.			
We celebrate successes achieved through data-driven marketing approaches.			
I am staying informed about emerging trends in marketing technologies and data analytics tools.			
I am committed to continuous improvement and adapting my marketing strategy based on ongoing data and performance analysis.			

9

THE FUTURE OF HEALTHCARE MARKETING: EMBRACING CONTINUOUS LEARNING

Welcome to Chapter 9, where we delve into the exciting and dynamic realm of emerging trends in AI and technology that are shaping the future of healthcare marketing. As a doctorpreneur, staying ahead of the curve and embracing continuous learning are crucial to thriving in this ever-evolving landscape.

STAYING AHEAD OF THE CURVE: EMERGING TRENDS IN AI AND TECHNOLOGY

Let's explore key areas that hold immense potential for transforming your marketing efforts:

1. Artificial Intelligence (AI) for Personalized Marketing:

   - AI-powered patient segmentation: Achieve hyper-personalization by segmenting patients based on demographics, health data, and behavioral patterns.

   - Dynamic content generation: Tailor marketing messages and recommendations to individual patient needs and preferences using AI-powered content creation tools.

   - Chatbots for patient engagement: Leverage AI-powered chatbots to provide 24/7 support, answer frequently asked questions, and schedule appointments.

- Predictive analytics: Anticipate patient needs and proactively offer relevant services or educational content through AI-driven insights.

- AI-powered sentiment analysis: Gauge patient sentiment towards your practice and marketing efforts through social media and online review analysis.

2. Augmented Reality (AR) and Virtual Reality (VR) for Immersive Experiences:

- AR-powered consultations: Offer virtual consultations and remote examinations using AR technology to enhance patient engagement and accessibility.

- VR simulations for patient education: Provide immersive and interactive learning experiences about health conditions and treatment options through VR.

- Interactive virtual tours: Showcase your practice facilities and equipment using VR tours, offering patients a glimpse into your environment.

- AR-enhanced marketing materials: Create engaging and interactive brochures, flyers, and other marketing materials with AR elements.

3. Blockchain for Secure and Transparent Data Management:

- Secure patient data storage and sharing: Utilize blockchain technology to securely store and share patient data with authorized individuals, ensuring privacy and transparency.

- Trackable supply chain management: Monitor the origin and movement of medical supplies and pharmaceuticals, enhancing safety and traceability.

- Improved patient engagement with medical records: Empower patients with secure access and control over their medical records through blockchain-based platforms.

4. Voice Search and Smart Assistants for Convenient Interactions:

   - Optimize for voice search: Ensure your website and marketing materials are optimized for voice search queries, increasing patient accessibility.

   - Develop skills for smart assistants: Create skills for popular smart assistants like Alexa or Google Assistant, allowing patients to book appointments, ask questions, and access information hands-free.

   - Offer voice-activated patient portals: Enable patients to manage appointments, access medical records, and communicate with your practice through voice commands.

5. Continued Evolution of Telehealth and Remote Care:

   - Expand telehealth offerings: Utilize telehealth for consultations, follow-up appointments, and remote monitoring to provide convenient access to care.

   - Develop patient education platforms: Create online platforms or mobile apps to deliver educational content, manage chronic conditions, and offer remote patient support.

   - Integrate telehealth with AI and other technologies: Combine telehealth with AI-powered chatbots, virtual assistants, and other tools to enhance patient experience and outcomes.

Remember: Embracing these emerging trends requires ongoing learning, adaptability, and a willingness to experiment. Start small, identify technologies that align with your goals and resources, and continuously evaluate their impact on your marketing effectiveness.

By staying informed, exploring new possibilities, and actively learning, you can position yourself as a forward-thinking doctorpreneur, leverage the power of technology to enhance your marketing, and build a thriving practice in the ever-evolving healthcare landscape.

ONGOING LEARNING RESOURCES FOR DOCTORPRENEURS

As a doctorpreneur, staying ahead of the curve in healthcare marketing necessitates continuous learning and exploration of new trends, technologies, and best practices. Here are some valuable resources to support your lifelong learning journey:

1. Industry Publications and Blogs:

   - Healthcare marketing blogs: Subscribe to blogs from leading healthcare marketing agencies, consultants, and industry publications like Medical Marketing & Media, Healthcare IT News, and The Healthcare Marketer.

   - Medical journals and publications: Stay updated on advancements in your medical field by subscribing to relevant journals and publications.

   - Technology and business publications: Follow publications like Harvard Business Review, Forbes, and Fast Company for broader business and technology insights.

2. Podcasts and Webinars:

   - Healthcare marketing podcasts: Listen to podcasts like Healthcare Marketing Lab, Healthcare Marketing Hustle, and The Doctors' Channel to gain insights from experts and industry leaders.

   - Live and on-demand webinars: Attend or stream webinars on various healthcare marketing topics offered by associations, platforms, and educational institutions.

   - Free online courses and tutorials: Take advantage of free online courses on platforms like Coursera, Udemy, and EdX covering diverse healthcare marketing topics, digital marketing skills, and technology trends.

3. Professional Organizations and Conferences:

   - Join industry associations: Become a member of relevant associations like the American Marketing Association (AMA) or the Healthcare Information and Management Systems Society (HIMSS) to access resources, events, and networking opportunities.

   - Attend healthcare marketing conferences: Participate in national or regional healthcare marketing conferences to learn from experts, network with peers, and discover new technologies.

- Connect with online communities: Join online communities and forums dedicated to healthcare marketing for peer support, discussions, and knowledge sharing.

4. Books and Ebooks:

- Invest in relevant books and ebooks: Stay updated on industry trends and best practices by reading books and ebooks authored by renowned healthcare marketing experts.

- Explore audiobooks and summaries: Utilize audiobooks and summaries for convenient learning on the go while commuting or during downtime.

- Join book clubs or discussion groups: Engage in active learning and discussion with peers by joining book clubs or online forums focused on healthcare marketing books.

5. Educational Platforms and Certifications:

- Enroll in online marketing courses: Pursue online certification programs or specialized courses focusing on healthcare marketing, digital marketing, or relevant technology areas.

- Seek mentorship opportunities: Connect with experienced healthcare marketing professionals for guidance, mentorship, and practical industry insights.

- Participate in workshops and training sessions: Enhance your skills through targeted workshops and training sessions on specific marketing tools, tactics, or emerging technologies.

Remember: The key is to be proactive, identify learning resources that align with your interests and goals, and dedicate time to consistent learning and skill development. Utilize a combination of different resources to create a well-rounded learning experience and adapt your approach as your needs and the industry evolve.

Share your thoughts! What are your favorite resources for ongoing learning and staying updated in the field of healthcare marketing?

By investing in your knowledge and skills through continuous learning, you can unlock your full potential as a doctorpreneur, navigate the dynamic healthcare landscape with confidence, and achieve sustainable success in your marketing endeavors.

BUILDING A SUSTAINABLE GROWTH STRATEGY FOR YOUR PRACTICE

As a doctorpreneur, achieving long-term success hinges on building a sustainable growth strategy for your practice. This goes beyond simply attracting new patients; it's about fostering loyalty, building strong relationships, and ensuring your practice thrives in the ever-evolving healthcare landscape. In this topic, we'll explore key elements to consider when building a sustainable growth strategy:

1. Define Your Unique Value Proposition:

    *   What makes your practice different and special? Identify your unique strengths, expertise, patient experience, or approach that sets you apart from competitors.

    *   Clearly articulate your value proposition: Clearly communicate what sets you apart and why patients should choose you. Incorporate it into your marketing materials, website, and patient interactions.

    *   Align your value proposition with your target audience: Ensure your value proposition resonates with the specific needs and preferences of your ideal patient demographic.

2. Focus on Patient Retention and Loyalty:

    *   Deliver exceptional patient care: Prioritize high-quality care, patient satisfaction, and positive experiences to keep patients coming back.

    *   Invest in patient relationships: Build trust and rapport with patients through personalized communication, active listening, and addressing their concerns effectively.

    *   Offer loyalty programs and incentives: Reward loyal patients with exclusive benefits, discounts, or special offers to encourage repeat business and advocacy.

3. Leverage Technology and Automation:

   - Streamline administrative tasks: Utilize technology to automate appointment scheduling, billing, and other administrative tasks, freeing up your time to focus on patient care.

   - Embrace telehealth and remote care: Offer telehealth options for consultations, follow-up appointments, and remote monitoring to enhance accessibility and convenience for patients.

   - Utilize data analytics: Leverage data insights to understand patient behavior, identify areas for improvement, and personalize your marketing and outreach efforts.

4. Diversify Your Services and Revenue Streams:

   - Explore new service offerings: Consider expanding your service portfolio to cater to unmet needs in your community or offer specialized services that align with your expertise.

   - Develop ancillary products or resources: Offer educational materials, online courses, or other products related to your field to generate additional revenue streams.

   - Collaborate with other healthcare providers: Partner with complementary practitioners to offer integrated care services and expand your reach.

5. Foster a Culture of Continuous Improvement:

   - Seek and embrace feedback: Actively solicit patient feedback through surveys, reviews, and direct communication to identify areas for improvement.

   - Invest in team development: Provide opportunities for your staff to learn new skills, attend training programs, and stay updated on industry advancements.

   - Monitor industry trends and adapt: Regularly evaluate the healthcare landscape, emerging technologies, and patient preferences to adapt your strategy and remain competitive.

Remember: Building a sustainable growth strategy is an ongoing process, not a one-time event. Regularly assess your progress, adapt your approach based on data and feedback, and be willing to experiment with new strategies to ensure your practice thrives in the long run.

By focusing on these key elements and fostering a culture of continuous learning and adaptation, you can build a thriving practice that delivers exceptional patient care, generates sustainable growth, and positions you for success in the ever-evolving healthcare landscape.

UNLEASHING THE POWER OF WHATSAPP: MARKETING AND PATIENT RELATIONS FOR DOCTORS

In today's digitally connected world, patients expect convenient and personalized communication with their healthcare providers. WhatsApp, with its massive user base and user-friendly interface, presents a unique opportunity for doctors to bridge the gap and enhance both marketing and patient relations. This chapter delves into the world of WhatsApp marketing for healthcare, empowering doctors to leverage its potential for growth and improved patient engagement.

WHY WHATSAPP FOR DOCTORS?

Compared to traditional communication channels, WhatsApp offers several advantages for doctors:

- High User Penetration: With over 2 billion active users globally, WhatsApp boasts a wider reach than most marketing platforms, ensuring your message reaches your target audience.

- Direct Communication: Unlike emails, WhatsApp messages land directly on patients' phones, enabling real-time communication and fostering a sense of immediacy.

- Personalized Engagement: Features like groups, broadcast lists, and individual chats allow for tailored communication based on patient needs and preferences.

- Convenience and Accessibility: Patients can easily access information and connect with you at their convenience, eliminating geographical barriers and time constraints.

- Cost-Effectiveness: Compared to traditional marketing methods, WhatsApp offers a cost-effective solution for promoting your practice and services.

MARKETING YOUR PRACTICE WITH WHATSAPP:

- Create a Profile: Build a professional WhatsApp Business profile highlighting your expertise, services, and contact information.

- Offer Value-Added Content: Share informative and engaging content like health tips, appointment reminders, and educational videos to attract new patients.

- Targeted Broadcasts: Send informative messages to groups based on specific demographics or health conditions, promoting relevant services and special offers.

- Offer Chat Support: Utilize the chat function to answer patient queries, clarify doubts, and address concerns in real-time, enhancing patient satisfaction.

- Leverage Interactive Features: Utilize features like polls and quizzes to encourage engagement and gather valuable patient insights.

- Run Contests and Giveaways: Organize interactive contests and giveaways to attract new followers and promote specific services.

BUILDING STRONGER PATIENT RELATIONSHIPS:

- Appointment Reminders and Confirmations: Send automated appointment reminders and confirmations to reduce no-shows and improve patient punctuality.

- **Post-Consultation ** Use WhatsApp to check in with patients after appointments, answer questions, and address any concerns.

- Telemedicine Consultations: Utilize WhatsApp video calls for remote consultations, offering convenient care options for patients unable to visit in person.

- Group Support Chats: Create support groups for patients with specific conditions to facilitate peer-to-peer interaction and promote emotional well-being.

- Share Educational Resources: Send patients relevant articles, brochures, and educational videos to empower them to actively participate in their healthcare journey.

- Personalized Communication: Utilize individual chats to address patient concerns with empathy and personalized guidance, fostering trust and loyalty.

IMPORTANT CONSIDERATIONS:

- Privacy and Security: Ensure strict adherence to patient data privacy regulations and utilize WhatsApp's built-in security features.

- Professionalism: Maintain a professional tone in all communications, avoiding informal language or self-promotion.

- Responsiveness: Aim for prompt responses to messages, demonstrating respect for patients' time and concerns.

- Consent and Opt-Out: Obtain explicit consent from patients before adding them to groups or broadcast lists, and provide clear opt-out options.

By embracing WhatsApp marketing and integrating it into patient communication strategies, doctors can:

- Reach a wider audience and attract new patients.

- Enhance patient engagement and build stronger relationships.

- Improve appointment adherence and follow-up care.

- Offer convenient and accessible healthcare services.

- Ultimately, contribute to better patient outcomes and a more fulfilling practice.

Remember, the key to success lies in using WhatsApp responsibly, ethically, and strategically. By leveraging its potential for communication and connection, doctors can create a thriving practice centered on patient care and satisfaction.

SUMMARY

- AI for personalized marketing: patient segmentation, dynamic content, chatbots, predictive analytics, sentiment analysis.

- AR/VR for immersive experiences: virtual consultations, patient education, interactive tours, AR-enhanced marketing materials.

- Blockchain for secure data management: secure storage, trackable supply chain, improved patient engagement with records.

- Make scope for voice search and smart assistants on your web portal, develop voice search optimization, skills for smart assistants, voice-activated patient portals.

- Continued evolution of telehealth and remote care: expanded telehealth offerings, patient education platforms, integration with AI.

- Industry publications and blogs, podcasts and webinars, free online courses, professional organizations and conferences, books and ebooks, educational platforms and certifications.

- Be proactive, identify relevant resources, dedicate time to consistent learning, adapt your approach as needed.

- Define your unique value proposition, focus on patient retention and loyalty, leverage technology and automation.

- Diversify your services and revenue streams, foster a culture of continuous improvement.

- Regularly assess progress, adapt your approach, and be willing to experiment.

SELF ASSESSMENT CHECKLIST

Questions	Yes	No	Notes
I am aware of emerging trends in AI and technology that are shaping the future of healthcare marketing.			
I am actively exploring how these trends could be applied to my marketing strategy.			
I am comfortable experimenting with new technologies and adapting my approach based on results.			
I have identified resources for staying updated on the latest trends in healthcare marketing.			
I dedicate time each week or month to learning and professional development.			
I am actively building my knowledge and skills in relevant areas like digital marketing, data analytics, and emerging technologies.			
I have a clearly defined unique value proposition that sets my practice apart.			
I am actively building strong relationships and fostering loyalty among my patients.			
I am leveraging technology and automation to streamline processes and improve efficiency.			
I am exploring ways to diversify my services and revenue streams.			
I am committed to continuous improvement and adapting my strategy based on data and feedback.			

BONUS CHAPTER

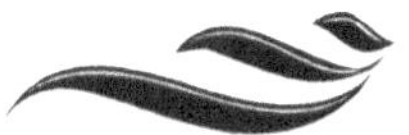

CASE STUDIES: DOCTORPRENEURS WHO CRACKED THE AI CODE

In this bonus chapter, we delve into the inspiring journeys of doctorpreneurs who have successfully leveraged AI in their marketing strategies, achieving remarkable results and paving the way for the future of healthcare marketing. Through these real-world examples, you'll gain valuable insights and practical inspiration to implement AI in your own practice:

CASE STUDY 1: DR. AMAN VOKENDI- PERSONALIZED APPOINTMENT REMINDERS WITH AI CHATBOT

Challenge: Dr. Aman, a practicing Gastroenterologist from Kota, faced high appointment no-show rates, impacting patient care and revenue. Traditional reminder methods proved ineffective.

Solution: He implemented an AI-powered chatbot that sends personalized appointment reminders via text message. The chatbot engages in two-way conversations, answering patient questions, confirming appointments, and offering rescheduling options.

Results: Appointment no-show rates reduced by 30%, saving time and resources, while patient satisfaction increased due to convenient and personalized communication.

KEY LEARNINGS:

- AI chatbots can automate tasks, improve communication, and enhance patient experience.

- Personalization is key: tailor AI interactions to individual patient needs and preferences.

CASE STUDY 2: DR. KUSUM SHARMA - AI-DRIVEN CONTENT MARKETING FOR PATIENT EDUCATION

Challenge: Dr. Kusum ,a Homeopath from Pune struggled to create engaging and informative content for his website and social media, limiting patient reach and education.

Solution: She adopted an AI content creation platform that analyzes her medical expertise and patient data to generate personalized health articles, blog posts, and social media content.

Results: Website traffic increased by 50%, and patient engagement with educational content significantly improved. This led to a rise in appointment bookings and patient referrals.

KEY LEARNINGS:

- AI can create high-quality, relevant content at scale, saving time and resources.

- Data-driven content resonates with patients and fosters trust and engagement.

CASE STUDY 3: DR. KUMUD RAJAGOPALACHARI - AI-POWERED PATIENT SEGMENTATION FOR TARGETED MARKETING

Challenge: Dr. Kumud Rajagopalachari, a dentist from Chennai was facing the challenge that marketing efforts lacked focus, reaching a broad audience with generic messages, resulting in low conversion rates.

Solution: He set with his digital marketing agency to get the real data and statistics from tools like Google Adwords and Facebook of his patients. The agency also used an AI-powered patient segmentation tool that analyzes patient demographics, medical history, and engagement data to create targeted patient segments.

Results: By tailoring marketing messages and campaigns to specific patient segments, Dr. Kumud achieved a 20% increase in conversion rates for appointments and consultations.

KEY LEARNINGS:

- AI-powered segmentation helps identify ideal patients and personalize marketing efforts.

- Targeted campaigns with relevant messaging resonate better and drive higher engagement.

Bonus Tip: Remember, AI is a powerful tool, but ethical considerations are paramount. Ensure transparency, data privacy, and responsible use of AI in your marketing strategy.

These are just a few examples of how doctorpreneurs are leveraging AI to transform their marketing and achieve success. As you explore these case studies, consider how you can adapt and implement similar strategies in your own practice to unlock the potential of AI and thrive in the ever-evolving healthcare landscape.

INSIGHTS AND TAKEAWAYS TO INSPIRE YOUR OWN JOURNEY

As we reach the conclusion of this exploration, let's take a moment to reflect on the key insights and takeaways that can empower you on your own doctorpreneur journey. Remember, the path to success is paved with continuous learning, adaptation, and a willingness to embrace the future. Here are some valuable gems to carry with you:

1. Stay Ahead of the Curve:

   - Embrace lifelong learning: Dedicate time to learning about emerging trends, technologies, and best practices in healthcare marketing.

   - Explore AI and other innovations: Be open to experimenting with new tools and approaches to differentiate your practice and enhance patient experience.

   - Seek inspiration from others: Learn from the successes and challenges of fellow doctorpreneurs and adapt their strategies to your unique context.

2. Build Strong Patient Relationships:

   - Focus on personalization: Tailor your marketing messages and approach to individual patient needs and preferences.

   - Invest in patient communication: Prioritize clear, effective, and two-way communication to build trust and loyalty.

   - Foster a culture of care: Go beyond medical expertise and create a welcoming, supportive environment for your patients.

3. Leverage Technology Strategically:

   - Identify areas for automation: Streamline administrative tasks and free up your time for patient-centered activities.

   - Embrace telehealth and remote care: Offer convenient and accessible care options to meet evolving patient needs.

   - Utilize data analytics: Gain insights from patient data to inform your marketing decisions and improve patient outcomes.

4. Cultivate a Growth Mindset:

   - Set SMART goals: Define clear, measurable, achievable, relevant, and time-bound goals for your practice.

- Track your progress: Regularly monitor your marketing efforts and measure the impact of your strategies.

- Be adaptable and agile: Embrace change, experiment with new ideas, and readily adapt your approach based on results and feedback.

5. Remember the Human Touch:

- Technology is a tool, not a replacement: While technology can enhance your practice, never lose sight of the importance of human connection and empathy.

- Prioritize patient care: At the heart of it all, your success hinges on delivering exceptional medical care and building meaningful relationships with your patients.

- Find your unique voice: Authentically represent your expertise, values, and passion in your marketing efforts to connect with patients on a deeper level.

Remember, the journey of a doctorpreneur is never-ending. Embrace the challenges, celebrate the successes, and keep learning, growing, and adapting. By incorporating these insights and takeaways into your approach, you can navigate the ever-evolving healthcare landscape with confidence, build a thriving practice, and make a lasting impact on the lives of your patients.

Appendix: Additional Resources and Tools for Doctorpreneurs

This appendix provides a curated list of valuable resources and tools to support your journey as a doctorpreneur, categorized for easy access:

1. Ongoing Learning and Development:

   - Industry Publications and Blogs:

     - Healthcare Marketing & Media: https://www.floridatechonline.com/blog/healthcare-management/healthcare-marketing-definition-and-job-outlook/

     - Medical Marketing and Media: https://www.mmm-online.com/

     - Healthcare IT News: https://www.healthcareitnews.com/

     - The Doctors' Channel: https://www.thedoctorschannel.com/

     - Practo Health Wiki : https://www.practo.com/health-wiki

   - Podcasts and Webinars:

     - Healthcare Marketing Lab: https://podcasts.feedspot.com/healthcare_marketing_podcasts/

     - Healthcare Marketing Hustle: https://www.thehealthcarehustlepodcast.com/

     - The Doctors' Channel Podcasts: https://www.thedoctorschannel.com/

- American Marketing Association (AMA) Webinars: https://www.ama.org/ama-advertising-hub/webinars/

- Online Courses and Platforms:

  - Coursera: https://www.coursera.org/courses?query=healthcare

  - Udemy: https://www.udemy.com/

  - EdX: https://www.edx.org/

  - AMA Marketing Certifications: https://www.ama.org/training-for-marketing/

2. Technology and Automation:

   - Telehealth Platforms:

     - Practo Consult: https://www.practo.com/consult/ :

     - For Hospitals: https://www.practo.com/providers/hospitals/insta

     - Lybrate: https://www.lybrate.com/

     - DocsApp: https://www.docsapp.in/

     - Teladoc Health: https://www.teladochealth.com/

     - Amwell: https://business.amwell.com/

     - Doctor.com: https://www.doctor.com/search

   - Appointment Scheduling and Patient Engagement Tools:

     - Zocdoc: https://www.zocdoc.com/

     - Healthgrades: https://www.healthgrades.com/

     - Kareo: https://www.kareo.com/

   - Data Analytics and Marketing Automation Platforms:

     - HubSpot: https://www.hubspot.com/

     - Mailchimp: https://mailchimp.com/

     - Constant Contact: https://www.constantcontact.com/

     - Google Analytics: https://marketingplatform.google.com/about/analytics/

3. Building a Sustainable Growth Strategy:

   - Patient Relationship Management (PRM) Systems:

     - Zoho CRM: https://www.zoho.com/crm/

     - Salesforce Health Cloud: https://www.salesforce.com/products/health-cloud/overview/

     - Microsoft Dynamics 365 Customer Service: https://learn.microsoft.com/en-us/dynamics365/customer-service/implement/overview

   - Patient Education and Content Creation Platforms:

     - Sharecare: https://www.sharecare.com/

     - WebMD: https://www.webmd.com/

     - PatientsLikeMe: https://www.patientslikeme.com/

   - Professional Organizations and Communities:

     - American Marketing Association (AMA): https://www.ama.org/

     - Healthcare Information and Management Systems Society (HIMSS): https://www.himss.org/

     - American Medical Association (AMA): https://www.ama-assn.org/

     - The Society for Healthcare Strategy and Market Development (SHSMD): https://www.shsmd.org/

4. Staying Informed about AI and Emerging Trends:

   - Industry Reports and Whitepapers:

     - McKinsey & Company: https://www.mckinsey.com/

     - Accenture: https://www.accenture.com/us-en

     - Harvard Business Review: https://hbr.org/the-latest

- AI in Healthcare Conferences and Events:

  - HIMSS Conference & Exhibition: https://www.himss.org/

  - The Healthcare AI Summit: https://boston-ai-healthcare.re-work.co/

  - The AI in Healthcare Symposium: https://online.stanford.edu/programs/artificial-intelligence-healthcare

- AI in Healthcare Podcasts and Blogs:

  - The Health AI Podcast: https://open.spotify.com/show/1o2edNIXTHZCiv0RmfMnlL

  - Healthcare Data Science: https://podcasts.apple.com/us/podcast/healthcare-data-matters-podcast/id1541382920

  - Singularity Hub: https://singularityhub.com/

5. Remember:

   - This list is not exhaustive, and new resources emerge frequently. Explore and find what works best for you.

   - Utilize a combination of resources to gain diverse perspectives and well-rounded knowledge.

   - Stay dedicated to continuous learning and adapt your approach as the healthcare landscape evolves.

By leveraging these valuable resources and tools, you can empower yourself to thrive as a doctorpreneur, build a successful practice, and make a positive impact on the healthcare ecosystem.

Glossary of Terms for Doctorpreneurs

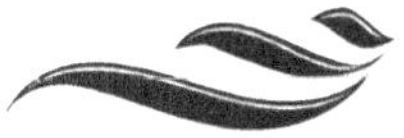

AI (Artificial Intelligence): The ability of machines to mimic human cognitive functions like learning and problem-solving. In healthcare, AI can be used for tasks like diagnosis, treatment planning, and drug discovery.

API (Application Programming Interface): A set of tools and protocols that allows different software applications to communicate and exchange data.

Blockchain: A secure, distributed ledger technology that can be used to track and record transactions transparently and immutably.

Data Analytics: The process of collecting, cleaning, and analyzing data to extract insights and inform decision-making.

Digital Marketing: Marketing using digital channels like websites, social media, and email.

Healthcare IT (HIT): The use of information technology in healthcare to improve efficiency, accuracy, and patient care.

Patient Relationship Management (PRM): Software that helps healthcare providers manage patient data, communication, and appointments.

Telehealth: The use of telecommunications technology to provide healthcare services remotely.

Telemedicine: The practice of diagnosing and treating patients remotely using telecommunications technology.

Teleconsultation: A consultation between a doctor and a patient that takes place remotely, typically using video conferencing.

Telemonitoring: The remote monitoring of a patient's health status using devices like wearable sensors.

Unique Value Proposition (UVP): What makes your practice different and special compared to competitors.

SOCIAL MEDIA MARKETING:

- Algorithm: The set of rules that social media platforms use to determine what content users see in their feeds.

- Engagement: The number of likes, comments, shares, and other interactions your content receives.

- Follower: A user who has subscribed to your social media page and sees your updates in their feed.

- Hashtag: A keyword or phrase preceded by # that helps users discover content related to a specific topic.

- Influencer: A person with a large following on social media who can promote your brand or product.

- Organic Reach: The number of people who see your content without paid promotion.

- Paid Advertising: Using paid options on social media platforms to reach a wider audience.

- Social Listening: Monitoring online conversations to understand what people are saying about your brand or industry.

- Social Proof: Positive reviews, testimonials, and social media engagement that demonstrate the value of your product or service.

LEAD FUNNELS:

- Lead: A potential customer who has shown interest in your product or service.

- Lead Magnet: A free offer, like an ebook or webinar, that entices users to share their contact information.

- Landing Page: A web page designed to capture leads, typically by offering a lead magnet in exchange for contact information.

- Call to Action (CTA): A clear instruction telling users what you want them to do next, such as "Download Now" or "Subscribe Here."

- Conversion Rate: The percentage of leads who take a desired action, such as making a purchase or scheduling an appointment.

- Nurturing: Cultivating relationships with leads by providing valuable content and offers until they are ready to convert.

- Drip Email Marketing: A series of automated emails sent to leads to educate them about your product or service and move them closer to conversion.

GOOGLE ADS:

- Keyword: A word or phrase that users type into search engines to find information.

- Keyword Research: Identifying relevant keywords that potential customers use to search for products or services like yours.

- PPC (Pay-Per-Click): An advertising model where you pay each time someone clicks on your ad.

- CPC (Cost-Per-Click): The average amount you pay for each click on your ad.

- CTR (Click-Through Rate): The percentage of people who see your ad and click on it.

- Quality Score: A Google Ads metric that assesses the relevance and quality of your keywords and landing page, impacting your ad ranking and cost.

- Ad Extensions: Additional information displayed with your ad, such as your address, phone number, or website links.

- Conversion Tracking: Measuring how many people who click on your ad take a desired action, such as making a purchase or contacting you.

- Remarketing: Targeting ads to users who have previously interacted with your website or app.

ADDITIONAL INDIAN-SPECIFIC TERMS:

- AYUSH: Ayurveda, Yoga, Unani, Siddha, and Homeopathy - the five traditional Indian systems of medicine.

- NHA (National Health Authority): The apex body responsible for implementing India's National Digital Health Mission (NDHM).

- ABHA (Ayushman Bharat Health Account): A unique digital health ID for every Indian citizen.

- EHR (Electronic Health Record): A digital version of a patient's medical history.

- PHC (Primary Health Center): The first point of contact for healthcare in rural India.

Remember: This glossary is not exhaustive and new terms emerge frequently. Stay updated on the latest developments in healthcare marketing and technology.

WOHOO, YOU'VE MADE IT

Congratulations, fellow doctorpreneurs! You've reached the end of this journey, equipped with a roadmap to navigate the exciting world of healthcare marketing and technology. By now, you possess a treasure trove of strategies and insights to attract patients, build loyalty, and ultimately, deliver exceptional care.

But remember, this is just the beginning. The healthcare landscape is constantly evolving, demanding agility and continuous learning. As you embark on your doctorpreneurship journey, keep these parting words in mind:

- Embrace the data-driven approach: Numbers don't lie. Leverage data analytics to measure, refine, and optimize your marketing efforts for maximum impact.

- Stay curious and experiment: Don't be afraid to try new things and learn from your experiences. Innovation is key to staying ahead of the curve.

- Focus on building relationships: Marketing goes beyond acquiring patients; it's about nurturing trust and loyalty. Connect with your audience on a human level.

- Never stop learning: Dedicate time to expanding your knowledge and staying updated on the latest trends in healthcare marketing and technology.

Remember, you're not alone on this path. If you're looking to accelerate your growth and unlock the full potential of your practice, I'm here to help. My expertise in healthcare marketing and growth hacking can guide you towards achieving your goals.

Ready to take your doctorpreneur journey to the next level?

Reach out to me at rishiaacharya82@gmail.com and let's discuss how I can tailor my professional services to your specific needs. Thank you for joining me on this journey. I wish you all the best in your doctorpreneurship endeavors!

Sincerely,

Dr. Rishi Aacharya

Growth Hacking Consultant for Healthcare Industry

SPECIAL GIFT

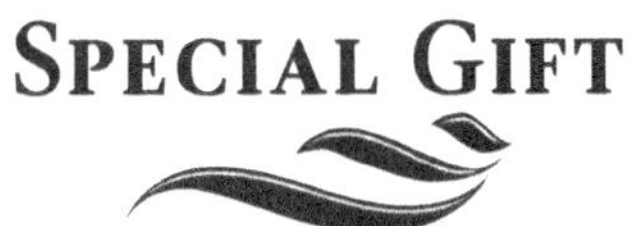

Book a 30 min one to one video call with me and see how you can grow your Healthcare Business by 10x in the next 3 months.

For appointment please write to me on rishiaacharya82@gmail.com

See you there.

9 798889 322299